T0177798

PSYCHOPHARMACOLOGY IN CANCER CARE

PSYCHOPHARMACOLOGY IN CANCER CARE

A Guide for Non-Prescribers and Prescribers

Andrew J. Roth, MD

Christian J. Nelson, PhD

OXFORD
UNIVERSITY PRESS

OXFORD
UNIVERSITY PRESS

Oxford University Press is a department of the University of Oxford. It furthers
the University's objective of excellence in research, scholarship, and education
by publishing worldwide. Oxford is a registered trade mark of Oxford University
Press in the UK and certain other countries.

Published in the United States of America by Oxford University Press
198 Madison Avenue, New York, NY 10016, United States of America.

CIP data is on file at the Library of Congress
ISBN 978-0-19-751741-3

DOI: 10.1093/med/9780197517413.001.0001

1 3 5 7 9 8 6 4 2

Printed by LSC Communications, United States of America

We dedicate this book to past, present, and future providers
of care for people with cancer and their families.

In memory of
Jimmie C. Holland
*A pioneering, dynamic, and humble woman who developed
the field of psycho-oncology and paved the way for this book*
Marguerite Lederberg
A teacher's teacher and a survivor

Both were master bridge builders and game changers.

CONTENTS

FOREWORD

When I was a graduate student in psychology many years ago, the first thing I learned was, "Before psychology, rule out biology." Drs. Andrew Roth and Christian Nelson have provided a much-needed road map for exactly how the non-prescribing clinician, in collaboration with the prescribing psychiatric–oncologist and/or physician, can usefully apply this principle. Now more than ever, with the focus on patient-centered care and patient-reported outcomes as central to quality cancer care, there is an urgency to educating clinicians and integrating neurobiology and psychology.

In the United States, more than 17 million people were diagnosed with cancer in 2019, and it is estimated that this number will increase to 27.5 million annual cases by 2040 due to population growth and aging, as well as advances in early detection and treatment.[1]

Along with the increase in overall cancer incidence, the number of people surviving cancer has also increased. Indeed, there are more than 16.9 million cancer survivors, and that number is projected to grow to more than 22.1 million by 2030.[2] Furthermore, with new tailored immunotherapies based on genomics and biomarkers, cancer is no longer treated as a monolithic disease. In fact, it is now understood to include a wide range of diseases for which targeted individualized care is fast becoming the norm. As a result, cancer treatment has become more complex, making it more difficult to comprehend all options and compare experiences with others. So, although improved clinical outcomes are being achieved for many patients (e.g., improved survival rates), the challenge to adapt to a cancer diagnosis, make treatment decisions, manage side effects of treatment and long-term survivorship issues, and, for some, confront death remains daunting.

Along with these trends in incidence and survival, we also find ourselves in an era in which four significant shifts are occurring in the health care delivery system in the United States and, specifically, in the patient experience. The primary forces for change are (1) the unsustainable cost of health care in the United States, estimated at $2.9 trillion annually, four-fifths of which is spent on 20% of the population who have complex medical disorders and chronic diseases such as diabetes, heart failure, and cancer; (2) the rise of the "engaged" patient coupled with the focus on a more patient-centered system of care;[3] (3) the mounting evidence that patient-reported outcomes (PROs) are an essential component of quality health care; and (4) due to the COVID-19 pandemic, the emergence of telehealth as an essential component of treatment.

Patient-centered care, the "blockbuster drug" of the 21st century, places the needs of patients and their family/caregivers at the center of the treatment approach. It differs from the traditional medical model, which focuses primarily on clinical outcomes such as tumor progression and survival rates. A growing body of research has shown that patient-centered care sets in motion increased engagement, which in turn leads to better experiences and outcomes.[4] Such improvements outstrip even the most successful drugs. Emerging evidence indicates that patient-centered care also reduces costs.[5] For cancer patients, there is considerable evidence of the benefits of social and emotional support on health.[6] In fact, understanding the patient experience moves beyond PROs and takes into account the broader context in which patients experience their disease and its consequences. It is inclusive of physical and emotional health, family and caregiver relationships, and personal goals and aspirations, including work and meaning in life.

These are all important theoretical frameworks for care. But how do these important goals become operationalized? Drs. Roth and Nelson—eminently qualified as clinicians, researchers, and practitioners—push the reader beyond the framework of non-prescribers versus prescribing clinicians and empirically delineate a collaborative model of care for psychology and psychiatry. Clearly written, *Psychopharmacology in Cancer Care* is a manual for integrative collaboration across disciples in psycho-oncology, psychotherapy, and psychopharmacology. This book underscores the hand-in-glove relationship between psychopharmacology and psychotherapy.

We understand that cancer can be a multiple traumatic event. The diagnosis, treatment, side effects and long-term consequences of treatment, threat of recurrence, and family and financial burden all create a complex palette from which the clinical and the prescribing teams must work together to differentiate biology from psychology. Moreover, as the authors underscore, oncologists and general medical practitioners most frequently prescribe psychiatric medications to their cancer patients. Yet, few oncology practices have dedicated psychiatric consultants familiar with the nuances of psycho-oncology. The non-prescribers' role is critical in helping patients identify "micro-improvements" due to medications. And, conversely, these practitioners can quickly note and differentiate side effects that are problematic and/or are transitory, thereby helping patients and families better regulate their anxiety and provide supportive care in an effort to "stay the course" as they exercise a degree of patience in the face of profound uncertainty.

In order to comprehend the importance of this book, we must place it in the context of the COVID-19 pandemic. The risk of even more fragmented care for oncology patients is profound. Their dreadful isolation and concomitant emotional distress continue to make headlines. With telehealth as a lifeline for care during this crisis, Drs. Roth and Nelson's guidance and wisdom are indispensable.

Mitch Golant, PhD, FAPOS

Clinical Psychologist

Fellow, American Psychosocial Oncology Society

Senior Consultant, Strategic Initiatives, Cancer Support

Community

NOTES

1. American Cancer Society. *Cancer treatment & survivorship facts & figures 2019–2021.* Atlanta, GA: American Cancer Society; 2019.
2. Cancer treatment and survivorship statistics.*CA Cancer J Clinicians* 2019 June;69(5). doi:10.3322/caac.21565.
3. Hibbard J, Greene J. What the evidence shows about patient activation: Better health outcomes and care experiences; Fewer data on costs. *Health Aff* 2013;32:2207–2214.
4. Kish L. The blockbuster drug of the century: An engaged patient. 2012. https://healthstandards.com/blog/2012/08/28/drug-of-the-century/. Accessed August 29, 2014.

5. National Research Council. *Best care at lower cost: The path to continuously learning health care in America.* Washington, DC: National Academies Press; 2013.

6. Gayer C, Buzaglo JS, Miller MF, Morris A, Kennedy V, Golant M. Meeting patient-centered standards: CancerSupportSource—A community-based distress screening program. *J Natl Compr Canc Netw* 2013;11(4):373–374.

ACKNOWLEDGMENTS

A wise person once suggested that some ideas needed to be written, but not everything written needs to be read.

This book has important information that will improve the lives of many people living with cancer. But what was originally written would not have been readable or digestible were it not for the gracious, conscientious editing by colleagues and friends who are expert in their own right. They gave generously of their time and knowledge and experience.

Mark Russ is a psychiatrist who is not a psycho-oncologist. He is the Vice Chair of Clinical Programs and Medical Director for New York Presbyterian/Cornell Westchester Psychiatry Program. His edits were vital for the optimal organization and presentation of our material. His decades of clinical, teaching, and writing experience helped clarify, correct, and redirect information that could otherwise lead non-prescribing clinicians astray or blind them to the pearls and potholes of our experience.

Allison Applebaum is an Assistant Attending Psychologist and Director of the Caregivers Clinic at the Department of Psychiatry and Behavioral Sciences at Memorial Sloan Kettering Cancer Center. She is not only an excellent clinician but also one who collaborates and communicates with prescribing psychiatrists and oncologists on a regular basis. A bonus for us is that she is a wonderful writer and a precise editor. She also recently edited an excellent book, *Cancer Caregivers*, published by Oxford University Press in 2019. Her comments helped shaped this book with suggestions a sculptor might use to chip away at granite to reveal a clearer and more meaningful message.

Rebecca Saracino is an Assistant Attending Psychologist in the Department of Psychiatry and Behavioral Sciences at Memorial Sloan Kettering Cancer Center, whose expertise in writing, and clinical acumen, far exceeds her years in practice. Her reading and edits of our manuscript facilitated a seamless transfer of our information to all non-prescribing clinicians. She made sure our information was detailed but relevant. Her smiley faces for the parts that worked were encouraging and uplifting.

Emily Kantoff is a pioneering Advanced Practice Nurse Practitioner in the Department of Psychiatry and Behavioral Sciences at Memorial Sloan Kettering Cancer Center who works as a psycho-oncology prescriber. Her editing for clarity, accuracy, and applicability helped connect the views and needs of non-prescribing clinicians and prescribers of all fields who may find themselves as the only psychotropic prescriber for a person with cancer. Her talents made our material clearer and more visually presentable.

Jeffrey Freedman is an Attending Psychiatrist at Memorial Sloan Kettering Cancer Center who has extensive experience in the field of consultation–liaison psychiatry and who has become a psycho-oncologist. His edits of our manuscript, gleaned from his proficiency as a seasoned Letter to the Editor contributor, helped us keep our facts straight and aided our translations from psycho-oncolog-ese to usefulness for clinicians of all backgrounds who find themselves caring for people with cancer.

Penelope Damaskos is the Director of Social Work at Memorial Sloan Kettering Cancer Center. She collaborates with clinicians in many areas of oncology and is a leader of integrated psychosocial care for people with cancer. Her spirited support early in our writing of this book was heartening and helpful.

Dianne Mead is a Clinical Social Worker at the Westchester Regional Ambulatory site of Memorial Sloan Kettering Cancer Center, whom Dr. Roth has the great fortune of working with on a weekly basis. Her humor and boundless energy encourage and guide colleagues and patients to better care and better health. Discussions with Dr. Roth over the course of the writing of this book helped the finished product remain pertinent and provided lucidity to otherwise complex information.

Nathan Kravis is a psychiatrist, teacher, and author who has been a priceless confidante to Dr. Roth for more than 30 years. He helped edit the course of Dr. Roth's life, so why not the manuscripts of his books? He is author of *On the Couch: A Repressed History of the Analytic Couch from Plato to Freud* (MIT Press, 2017).

Donna Greenberg is a psychiatrist in the Division of Psychiatry and Medicine at Massachusetts General Hospital who first invited Dr. Roth to participate in a half-day workshop on psychopharmacology in cancer care. She realized how much prescribers and non-prescribing clinicians needed basic psycho-oncology psychopharmacologic information.

We have since completed additional workshops and are appreciative that Dr. William Breitbart, Chairman of the Department of Psychiatry and Behavioral Sciences at Memorial Sloan Kettering Cancer Center, suggested an all-day seminar on this topic for all clinicians in cancer care, presented annually through the Memorial

Sloan Kettering Cancer Center's Psycho-Oncology Education and Training Institute. The experiences, lessons, and feedback from these workshops are what led our editor at Oxford University Press, Andrea Knobloch, to suggest we write this book. We are indebted to Andrea and Jacqueline Buckley for bringing this idea to reality.

We also acknowledge Dr. Steven Passik, who helped reshape Dr. Roth's early career thinking about which clinicians need to know about psychopharmacology. Dr. Passik is a psychologist whose expertise as a non-prescriber in cancer psychopharmacology shifted role perceptions among multidisciplinary cancer care providers, providing more integrated and comprehensive care of patients. Dr. Seema Thekdi, a psycho-oncologist in Houston, Texas, formerly of MD Anderson Cancer Center, was an organizer of an earlier version of our Psychopharmacology 101 conference and helped fine-tune our approach to teaching this material.

Dr. Roth has been fortunate to co-teach a class on Psychopharmacology in Cancer Care for the Fellowship Training Program at Memorial Sloan Kettering Cancer Center with Dr. Yesne Alici, Clinical Director of the Psychiatry Service. Dr. Alici's knowledge has provided important considerations for this book.

Dr. Roth feels blessed to have learned from and taught with Mitch Golant, PhD, a clinical psychologist and Senior Consultant for Strategic Initiatives for the Cancer Support Community and author of *What To Do When Someone You Love Is Depressed* (Holt Paperbacks, 2007) and Dr. Sherry R. Schachter, Executive Director Emerita of Bereavement Services at Calvary Hospital, whom he joined as faculty for a number of international psycho-oncology seminars that embodied optimal seamless interactions between prescribers and non-prescribers from hospital to community to end-of-life care. Their fun yet serious approach to teaching important and needed skills and proficiencies continues to be inspiring.

In addition, we thankfully acknowledge Nora Love, Dana Rathkopf, Tracy Curley, Julie Lowy, Katherine Kohrman, and Meyer Glaser, all superb clinicians from various specialties, who kindly offered to review parts of the manuscript; Howard Scher, Michael Morris, Susan Slovin, Daniel Danila, Christine Liebertz, and Gabrielle Arauz, who helped shape Dr. Roth's clinical acumen in real-time collaboration about the psychosocial and psychopharmacologic needs of people with cancer; Dr. Roth's supervisors and mentors at the Department of Psychiatry and Behavioral Sciences at Memorial Sloan Kettering, including Dr. Jimmie Holland, Dr. Marguerite Lederberg, Dr. Mary Jane Massie, Dr. William Breitbart, and Dr. Steven Passik; Ivy Belardo, a social worker with a heart of gold and many talents, who elevates the efforts of everyone with whom she works; and Michelle Ramsunder, Annie Kong, Sabina Bakar, and Kristen Kazanjian, who helped keep organizational order to Dr. Roth's daily work life so this book had the space and time to get written. Dr. Roth also acknowledges Rabbi Jeffrey Segelman for his wise encouragement to look beyond the cloak of illness to find the essence within and to recognize the interrelatedness of the spiritual, the psychological, and the physical.

Dr. Roth also acknowledges the memory of Dr. William Osler Benenson and Dr. Esther Siev Benenson, his parents-in-law, who modeled love of family, caring for others, and the integration of a multimodal approach to healing. Dr. Roth's parents Sherry and Albert set important examples of adjusting to adversity, working hard, and sacrificing for the benefit of others, while Dr. Roth's brother Jack has been a lifelong friend and inspiration to reach higher, care for the self, while helping others; he also modeled the art and faith of jumping into the adventures of authorship and putting unformed ideas to blank paper. Dr. Roth is enthusiastic about, and grateful for the current and future care providers in his life: his daughter Samara, a social worker who aids underprivileged and immigrant children and their families, and his son Bram, who has provided care and motivation to children with cancer and plans on a career in medicine. Finally, but not least, Dr. Roth is indebted to his wife Blanche (Bunny) Benenson, a pediatrician who has taught him so much about compassion for others and never giving up. She has inspired Dr. Roth's life and career for more than 40 years and enriches his ability to appreciate a more hopeful perspective on life as it develops.

We apologize for any inadvertent omissions in these acknowledgments. Any inconsistencies or incorrect information in this book are the sole responsibility of Dr. Roth and Dr. Nelson.

INTRODUCTION

I'm not a psycho-oncologist, and not even a prescriber—Why do
I need to know about psychiatric medications in cancer patients?

You may be asking yourself why you are holding this book about
psychopharmacology in the cancer setting in your hands right now,
even though you do not consider yourself a psycho-oncologist and
may have never even heard that term before. Maybe you are a social worker, a clinical psychologist or mental health counselor, a
registered or licensed practical nurse, a physical or occupational
therapist, a pharmacist, a chaplain or clergyperson, a research team
member, or even an administrative staff member who periodically
works with people who have cancer and observes their distress but
who cannot prescribe medications.

Or you are an advanced practice practitioner like a nurse practitioner, a physician assistant, a general medical practitioner, an
oncologist, or a psychiatrist who does not work primarily with
cancer patients but periodically sees such patients in your practice.
Psychiatric medications are most frequently prescribed to cancer

patients by oncologists and general medical practitioners because few oncology practices have dedicated psychiatric consultants familiar with the nuances of psycho-oncology. There is much overlap in the knowledge a prescriber needs to have in order to consider psychotropic medications in a medically healthy population, as well as in people with cancer. However, there are unique issues that practitioners should be aware of to better fine-tune treatments to a medically vulnerable population. Even when cancer patients receive psychotropic medications appropriately, they may have problems that arise before their next oncology visit or before they see the person who prescribed their psychiatric medications. Although prescribers are primarily responsible for managing these medications for patients, non-prescribing clinicians provide frontline psychosocial interventions and support for cancer patients. In doing so, they play an essential role in identifying psychological and physical symptoms, as well as detecting beneficial and problematic medication effects. We believe it is imperative for those who are not psycho-oncologists, or even prescribers, to have a place at the table of caring for people with cancer. Furthermore, even prescribers who are asked by patients for psychotropic medications are not obliged to concur or comply with those requests. We hope the information in this book will optimize proper referrals for medication assessment when appropriate, so patients have an important mechanism to improve the quality of their lives and get help to ameliorate their internal suffering.

The Institute of Medicine's 2008 report, *Cancer Care for the Whole Patient*,[1] highlighted barriers to identifying and addressing the psychosocial problems of patients. Inadequate communication between patients and prescribers, multiple demands on clinicians' time, and suboptimal coordination of care among providers due to a variety of local and systemic issues in the health care environment may all play a role in not adequately addressing these psychosocial needs, thus limiting cancer patients' quality of life. The stigma of suffering both a cancer diagnosis and psychological problems keeps providers and patients from more fully meeting these emotional needs. In addition to improving an individual's and/or family's quality of life, attention to emotional needs may enhance adherence with complicated cancer treatment regimens and, at times, help them cope better with adverse outcomes.

Non-prescribers are often the first responders to come in contact with the psychiatric distress of people with cancer. These clinicians have many skills at their disposal to deal with symptoms of depression, anxiety, and other quality-of-life sequelae of cancer and cancer treatment. Many nonmedication interventions, such as education, support, cognitive behaviorally oriented therapies, and other psychotherapies, as well as physical and occupational therapy, and spiritual guidance are offered or suggested by non-prescribers and may be sufficient to bring relief and improvement. But as we know, medications are also important treatments to manage many of these concerns. Non-prescribing clinicians can play an important role in helping patients best utilize psychotropic medication. You can help patients consider the best time to start a psychotropic intervention, educate patients to improve adherence to antidepressant treatment (i.e., the importance of daily dosing and how long it may take for the medication to work), and observe for potential side effects before a patient returns to see the psychotropic prescriber. As non-prescribers who understand the role of medications, you can be essential advocates for patients. Non-prescribing clinicians who understand the potential benefits of psychotropic medications can speed the referral of patients to qualified prescribers so problematic symptoms can be addressed, leading to improvement in adherence to, and tolerance of, cancer treatment. Non-prescribers do not need to be experts in surgery or the pharmacology of chemo-therapy. But knowledge of the medical and oncology factors that can cause reactions of anxiety or depression can help non-prescribers offer helpful insights to patients. This may decrease the likelihood that patients shun psychiatric care because they blame themselves for feeling "weak" or "weak-minded" or thinking that accepting psychiatric care indicates a moral weakness. Patients may experience emotions more intensely now that they have cancer. Families often feel emotions similar to those of patients, yet they may mask those emotions by portraying the opposite emotions to their loved one in attempts to cheer them up: "Don't worry, everything will be fine." (Silent response by patient: "Oh yeah, how do you know?") "The doctors are doing the best they can." (Silent response by patient: "Oh yeah, and what if that's not good enough? I will die."). Fear and sadness do not imply the patient has a psychiatric disorder or that a psychiatric medication is needed. All clinicians can watch out for inadvertent unhelpful communications that can hit a sore spot and lead to higher anxiety or lower mood: "You failed the treatment" as opposed to "The treatment did not work or failed you." "You don't qualify for the experimental protocol" is often heard as "I'm not good enough, or strong enough, or too sick." Here is where clinicians can provide crucial reframing, or healthier ways to view the situation.

Support and validation are essential psychotherapeutic devices when no psychotropic medications are needed; they may be even more important when there is a role for medications and the non-prescribing clinician has a clearer sense of how those medications fit into the overlapping arenas of oncology and mental health.

Dr. Roth has given many workshops on these topics for more than 10 years. He has received much feedback by non-prescribing clinicians and prescribers about what they want to learn and what they need to learn Dr. Nelson is a psychologist who has provided education, support and psychotherapy to patients with cancer and their families. He teaches non-prescribers how and when to refer patients for psychotropic medications and how to optimize psychotherapy and identify side effects that may occur when patients receive medications for psychiatric syndromes. They have worked together for 20 years developing strategies to bridge the psychopharmacologic gap between non-prescribers and prescribers in cancer care. For some, there will be much new information here. For others, it may feel like a review. Finding common ground for such a diversity of specialists and generalists is not easy or straightforward, but it is crucial for the emotional well-being of people with cancer. Our goal is to provide a road map with enough directions for non-prescribers and prescribers alike who care for people with cancer to improve pharmacologic treatment of distress, but not to get too bogged down with too many academic references. There is a suggested reading section at the end of the book for those who want to learn more.

A NON-PRESCRIBER'S PERSPECTIVE ON THE IMPORTANCE OF PSYCHOPHARMACOLOGY IN THE CANCER SETTING

Today, patients spend increasingly less time in examination rooms with those who may prescribe psychotropic medications. This book is written to bridge the supportive care/psychopharmacology gap between those who use various skills to address emotional and physical distress in people with cancer and those who prescribe psychotropic medication so that both will see patients with a more holistic perspective though their roles are distinct. We will teach you to supplement and enhance your essential clinical and observation skills to improve the quality of life, mental health, and safety of people you encounter with cancer.

THE ROAD MAP (A GUIDE TO THE GUIDE)

We cover five major topics of oncology psychopharmacology: antidepressants, anxiolytics, antipsychotics, medications for sleep disturbance, and medications for fatigue. Each chapter has a similar template, although for obvious reasons, one map cannot satisfy all topics. There will be road signs to help you find your way. We hope this road map will facilitate reading each chapter in its entirety or to more easily dive, or dip into, specific areas of interest.

In general, the template is as follows:

Introduction to the psycho-oncology syndrome and medications that may help

Risk factors and prevalence for psycho-oncology syndrome

Diagnostics: Accentuate the pearls, avoid the potholes

Symptoms

Algorithm for diagnosing

Medical look-alikes that can mask identification of the syndrome (consider other origins of symptoms)

Variables that may tip the prescriber to recommend a medication

Meds for heads: Get to know the names of medications to treat each syndrome

How the medications for this syndrome work: Myths and realities

Strategies prescribers use to choose appropriate medications

Benefits to hope for and the good and bad of side effects

Pearls and potholes that highlight potential deal-breaking side
effects of a particular medication in a particular situation

Safety considerations

Multitasking twofers: Solving a few problems with one
medication

Clinical cases are discussed throughout each chapter to highlight diagnostic or treatment pearls.

In addition, we developed a MedEscort Guide that will give you a sky view bottom-line description of the pertinent medications, and will spotlight essential information, treatment facts, and pearls and potholes. Communication guidelines that aid exchange of observations and information between non-prescribing clinicians and prescribers and may be vital to patient care and quality of life are reviewed. For example,

Q: What can non-prescribing clinicians do with regard to
psychopharmacology?

A: A great deal!

Well-informed non-prescribers can assist their patients in many ways when patients are considering taking or currently taking psychotropic medications. These medications may be essential to helping with the therapy strategies already being provided, whether psychological or medical. If the goal is to help the patient cope with their cancer diagnosis and treatment, optimizing the supportive care and psychotropic approaches are essential.

GENERAL THEMES

Discussions All Clinicians Can Have with Patients About Psychotropic Medications

At times, non-prescribing clinicians as well as non-psycho-oncology prescribers may be in the optimal position to discuss the potential importance of starting psychotropic medications with patients and family members. There are multiple topics all clinicians who care for people with cancer can utilize to promote patient education regarding psychotropic medications. Increased openness to having discussions to facilitate better understanding may improve patient cooperation and outcomes.

WHEN TO START PSYCHOTROPIC MEDICATIONS?

Because they interact with patients more frequently than do psycho-oncology prescribers, non-prescribing clinicians are well placed to assess and identify when psychotropic medications may be needed. We discuss when to refer a patient for psychotropic treatment and how to help the primary team monitor the patient for adverse effects, treatment response, and compliance. Non-prescribers will be better prepared to provide thoughtful psychoeducation to patients, family members, and oncology staff about when to consider a psychiatric medication and why now.

HOW DO THE MEDICATIONS WORK?

Readers will learn enough about how psychotropic medications work in cancer patients so that they can help patients make more informed decisions. Non-prescribers can help patients be more adherent to medication regimens by better grasping (1) how quickly, or slowly, a medication's beneficial effect is likely to start (onset of action); (2) how long the effect will generally last; (3) how often the medication should be taken in order to have its desired outcome and to avoid side effects; (4) how the medication should be taken (time of day; with or without food); and (5) when the medication could be discontinued by the prescriber.

ARE THERE USEFUL SIDE EFFECTS?

Readers will learn that some side effects may be very useful in a medically ill population. For example, drowsiness, an unwanted side effect during the day, can be helpful if the medication is taken at night for those who have trouble sleeping. Another side effect, weight gain, eschewed in a medically healthy person with depression, may be welcome in cancer patients who have lost their appetites, whether because of illness, cancer treatment, or depression. As non-prescribers learn more about which medications may provide "beneficial" side effects, they will be more prepared to discuss the possible benefits of these medications and provide better guidance on when to discuss starting a medication with a prescriber.

THE NOT-SO-USEFUL SIDE EFFECTS

Whether a patient with cancer receives a medication for anxiety, depression, confusion, insomnia, fatigue, nausea, or pain, the prescriber and others who care for the patient have an important opportunity to inform the patient and family (if appropriate) about possible side effects. Prior to prescribing a medication to a patient, Dr. Roth says,

> When I am considering taking a medication myself, I weigh the potential benefits against the potential side effects. Of course, the number of benefits listed in medication package inserts are

usually far fewer than the list of potential complications. But we know that most people will not get all of the problematic side effects, and many will get none.

Then we discuss the most common potential side effects, as well as the rare, but possibly dangerous, ones that many patients have heard about already (most likely from advertisements, such as the rare potential for antidepressants to cause suicidal ideation).

People with cancer may be less willing to accept quality-of-life impairment, such as fatigue or gastric upset, from a psychiatric medication than from those that may potentially save their lives, such as chemotherapy drugs. Although we all must assess our own acceptable risk versus benefit balance before taking any medication, we need useful information on which to make that decision. One important message to communicate to patients considering a psychotropic medication is that the *possibility* of getting a specific side effect is not necessarily a deal-breaking impediment, as even side effects of psychotropics can be managed. Another message is that non-prescribing caregivers can also detect the presence and intensity of side effects and determine what might be done to adapt to them, relieve them, and report them. Some side effects that arise early on after starting a medication commonly disappear after a few days or weeks so that the longer term benefit or goal can eventually outweigh the shorter term frustration of those side effects. Patients can also feel frustrated with themselves if they experience more intense side effects than their physicians predicted (e.g., nausea and fatigue). They might believe there is something wrong or deficient with them. At this point, it is important to let patients know that there is no "one size fits all" with regard to psycho-pharma-oncology, or any pharmacology. Our bodies do not read the "textbook" of how they are expected to respond, and that is why ongoing monitoring and surveillance by all providers is so important. Validation is a valuable nonpharmacologic intervention a non-prescriber can make about accepting or coping with medications or side effects. After cancer diagnoses, patients tend not to trust their bodies or their emotions as they did prior to cancer, as they may be in a period of shock or disbelief about the topsy-turvy flip their lives have taken. A non-prescribing clinician who is aware of psychopharmacology in cancer patients can help patients think about taking a medication to help mood, anxiety, or other symptoms and can help prescribers monitor patients for the not so good side effects before they lead to major problems or to non-adherence with a potentially valuable psychotropic medication.

"I DON'T WANT TO BECOME ADDICTED"

Often, patients (and non-prescribers) have misconceptions about psychotropic medications. One of these is the concern that people will become addicted to these medications. We discuss the potential of medication dependence, tolerance, addiction and withdrawal in the chapter on benzodiazepines and regarding pain medications such as opioids. Many patients are fearful of these controlled substances, often confusing the less likely phenomenon of "addiction" with the more common entities of "dependence" and "tolerance." We teach you strategies for screening patients with a higher likelihood of addiction and how you can help patients avoid tolerance when possible. Some patients will decide that the potential of addiction or tolerance is just not worth taking a medication because their symptom of pain or anxiety is not bad enough to justify the risk. It is also useful to acknowledge that cancer often steals a person's sense of control and autonomy. They may not believe they can refuse a cancer treatment suggestion to save their lives, but saying "no" to a psychotropic medication that they do not view as vital helps them maintain a sense of self-determination. However, without correct data, patients make decisions more from fear than from accurate information, and they will likely suffer worse quality of life than needed. Although addiction and misuse of these medications are possible, the risk:benefit ratio of using controlled substances may be different than in a general medical or psychiatric setting. Some medications are taken on an as needed (prn) basis. Others must be taken daily in order to build up a certain level over days or weeks before they will be effective. Taking a daily medication on a prn basis will make some people more susceptible to side effects, without any benefit of the good results. Similarly, a medication that should be taken as a prn that is instead taken daily may lead to ineffectiveness and perhaps dangerous side effects, dependence, or tolerance.

COMMUNICATING WITH THE PRIMARY TREATING TEAM

Non-prescribing clinicians will often see patients when the potential need for a psychotropic medication is just beginning. Sharing this information with the oncology team, or suggesting a referral to a psychiatric prescriber, can expedite a prescription and improvements in quality of life. The side effect profiles of psychotropic medications in people with cancer are like those in medically healthy people; however, the impact may be quite different depending on the influence the medication has on individual lifestyle and physiological circumstances. For instance, a person who is working a daytime job and needs to awaken early may be frustrated by a medication that leaves a groggy morning hangover effect. A healthy person struggling with weight issues may be less willing to accept a medication known to put on weight compared with a person with cancer who has been having appetite problems or nausea or weight loss.

Discussing your findings with the oncology team or prescriber can be vital. Your observations and follow-through may lead to more timely treatment for a patient who might otherwise suffer alone or in silence because they do not have the energy or the knowledge to pursue medications that may be helpful to them. In addition, cueing the prescriber about possible side effects that impair a patient's ability to function optimally can help recalibrate the patient's ability to navigate a rocky cancer landscape.

It is not unusual for patients to feel a degree of stigma or shame for having psychiatric symptoms such as depression or anxiety. They may feel embarrassed that they cannot tolerate a cancer regimen as well as they would want, or as they think their oncologist had hoped. Medical and psychological concerns overlap and impact each other in the world of cancer treatment. Patients may be embarrassed or scared to tell their oncologists that they are not handling things well, or that they dread possible side effects, for fear of appearing too weak to handle a lifesaving treatment. They may struggle with their self-identity of how strong they thought they were, or think they need to be, if they must "give in" and take pain medication or a medication to help them feel better emotionally. It is important to discuss with patients the safety and therapeutic reasons for communicating with all of their practitioners, and at times their family members, and to get the patients' approval. This type of information may be essential to better manage all of the medications the patient is receiving from multiple prescribers.

Do not assume that all the practitioners are getting the same picture. The patient's story may change based on how they have been feeling during the few days before seeing each practitioner. You, as the non-prescribing clinician, may have the best longitudinal view of the patient. You can emphasize the importance of team care and that you, the non-prescribing clinician, are part of that team, whether you are working in the same medical center, a different center, or in private practice.

Important Communication Bridges Non-Prescribers Can Have with Prescribers—Two Scenarios

I have been following your patient Ms. A for XYZ psychiatric issues for the past few weeks. She has worries about her cancer and treatment. I have found the following issues regarding her symptoms, which may or may not have to do with her medical treatment.

You can discuss any of the concerns you have, which may include the following:

- Medication adherence
- Abrupt cessation of anti-anxiety or pain medications and concerns about withdrawal
- Substance use or intoxication
- Using medications for multiple purposes (i.e., using lorazepam for anxiety instead of the nausea for which it was prescribed)
- Observations about a patient's symptoms such as difficulty sitting still, feeling a need to pace, social withdrawal, confusion, or unsteadiness while ambulating
- Information about side effects that may be related to the cancer or cancer treatment, such as urinary frequency, bowel incontinence, fatigue, pain, dizziness, difficulty walking, insomnia, nausea, loss of appetite, forgetfulness or cognitive slowing, or shakiness while writing or using utensils
- Suicidal ideation or passive thoughts of wanting to die because of sadness or demoralization about quality-of-life

problems such as pain or fatigue, cancer treatment issues, or inadequate social support. If the patient is actively suicidal with a plan or intent to hurt themselves, you will access emergency services immediately. Otherwise, you can collaborate with the primary treating providers to consider prescribing a psychotropic medication or adjusting a medication the patient is already on that might be contributing to the quality-of-life frustrations.

I have been following Mr. B for ABC psychiatric issues for the past few weeks. He does not attend therapy regularly, and when he does show up, he is unmotivated. He says he feels depressed most days, he doesn't sleep much because of anxiety about the future, and he feels hopeless about his cancer getting any better. I will continue to provide support, but I was hoping you could evaluate him for medications to improve his mood and sleep. He says he is embarrassed about telling you this; he is concerned that a psychiatric medication may make him ineligible for cancer treatment or may cause horrible side effects, and that just telling you he is not doing well will make him look weak in your eyes.

Helping Patients Take the Medications Correctly

Patients often get confused about what to do if they miss a dose or a few doses of a medication. Should they double up the next dose? Should they go back to an earlier dose if they have recently increased the dose? If they have skipped more than a few doses of the medication, whether because they were too nauseated to take the medication or because they forgot to take it, are they at risk for withdrawal from the medication? Prescribers are the appropriate providers to answer these questions; non-prescribers may not know all the answers, but they may be the first to hear the issues so can at least guide patients to have better communication with their prescribers. Patients who have financial constraints may halve medications in order to save money. This can be dangerous for some medications, depending on how long the patient had been on the prescribed dose. Decreasing doses below a therapeutic minimum can also reduce the potential usefulness of the medication. In fact, some medications will have more side effects if taken in lower doses (e.g., mirtazapine is more sedating in lower doses). If the non-prescriber does not listen for, and ask about these issues, they may not be addressed, and an important opportunity to facilitate better results may not be addressed.

Prescribers are often frustrated by patient noncompliance or non-adherence to medication regimes. This implies disobedience if a patient is not following the medication regimen exactly. It is possible, however, that the patient did not understand the instructions or otherwise was not able to tolerate the medication, feared possible side effects, or could not afford it. Before assuming someone is disobedient or not fully engaged in their treatment, we need to understand obstacles or concerns the patient may have had with following the prescribing instructions. Strategies that increase the likelihood of optimal implementation of prescribing instructions include writing down the instructions for taking the medication or giving patients preprinted information that is reviewed with them about how to take medications prescribed, as well as what possible side effects they might incur or read about in the medication package insert. It is helpful to have patients repeat back the suggested directions to ensure patients understand them. If the prescriber does not ask about questions, concerns or fears to be managed, this is a setup for failure that is really a communication failure. This is especially important for a patient who does not speak the same language as the prescriber. Because non-prescribers may have more time with a patient and understand some of their limitations, they may have a better sense that the medication will not be taken as prescribed. It may be because the patient's insurance will not cover the medication, the out-of-pocket outlay will be too expensive, the patient does not understand how to take it, or perhaps the patient does not believe in taking psychiatric medications. Helping the patient and prescriber attain a joint sense of understanding and partnership can be the missing piece of a puzzle of less than optimal medication adherence. Just because patients are able to navigate their care to a tertiary cancer center does not mean they have the resources to afford complete care.

BEFORE WE GET STARTED, SOME HOUSEKEEPING INFORMATION

(Prescribers may skip this section.)

The patient medical records you scrutinize will include abbreviations for various medication and prescribing nuances. Most health care providers develop prowess at recognizing and understanding this medical shorthand, although sometimes even they can misinterpret what was intended by another clinician. Much of this terminology derives from Latin, and some believe that this medical-ese was a covert attempt by doctors to keep a secret medical language from their patients. There will not be an exam at the end of this section, and you may not even see some of these terms in the book. But the sooner this code becomes familiar to you, the faster you will be able to focus on the essentials of helping your patients feel better. We also include some of own abbreviations that may be used in the book:

INTRODUCTION

AA = atypical antipsychotic such as olanzapine or quetiapine

ACh = anticholinergic

AD = antidepressant

ATC = around the clock; at regularly precribed hours; not 'as needed'

Benzo = benzodiazepine such as alprazolam, lorazepam, clonazepam, or diazepam

bid = twice a day (may be specified as every 12 hours)

BP = blood pressure

DC or D/C = discontinue

DDx = differential diagnosis (potential alternative diagnoses given a combination of symptoms)

DRI = dopamine reuptake inhibitor antidepressant

ECG = electrocardiogram

HR = heart rate

HS = at the hour of sleep; at bedtime

IV = intravenously

IM = intramuscularly

MAOI = monoamine oxidase inhibitor antidepressant

μg = microgram

mg = milligram

NRT = nicotine replacement treatment

OTC = over the counter

PO = per os; by mouth or orally

PR = per rectum; rectally

prn = as needed (in Latin this mean *pro re nata*, literally "for the thing born," but figuratively it means "as the circumstance arises" or "as needed")

q = every

q 2 h = every 2 hours

q 12 h = every 12 hours

qid = four times a day (may be specified as every 6 hours)

QOL = quality of life

Rx = prescription

SL = sublingually; under the tongue

SNRI = serotonin norepinephrine reuptake inhibitor antidepressants

SSRI = selective serotonin reuptake inhibitors (or serotonin-specific reuptake inhibitor) antidepressants

TCA = tricyclic antidepressant

tid = three times a day (may be specified as every 8 hours)

In each chapter, the following hand signal is used at various junctures:

This signal is strategically placed to indicate *stop and pay attention.* This sign emphasizes a pearl or pothole to be aware of. Although we think the whole book contains psycho-pharma-oncology pearls to follow and potholes to avoid, these hand signs highlight specific points we want to emphasize.

NOTE

1. Institute of Medicine. 2008. *Cancer care for the whole patient: Meeting psychosocial health needs.* NE Adler and AEK Page, eds. Washington, DC: National Academies Press.

Chapter 1

Antidepressants

INTRODUCTION

Depression is common in the general population. Major depression affects more than 17.3 million American adults, or approximately 7.1% of the US population aged 18 years or older, in a given year.[1] The prevalence of a depressive episode is higher among females (8.7%) compared with males (5.3%). Approximately 17–25% of people with cancer and other significant medical disorders will have symptoms suggestive of depression. The risk of depression plateaus from the ages of 65 to 75 years but then increases again with advancing age. Not everyone with depressive symptoms will have a major depressive episode, so it is important to recognize and address subsyndromal depression that could cause suffering and eventually lead to a clinically debilitating depressive episode. The most common diagnosis in people with cancer who have depressive symptoms is adjustment disorder. Alternatively, just because someone has a current or past major depressive episode does not mean they do not also have a different psychiatric disorder that needs to be addressed now. Many people with cancer who have major depression will also have accompanying anxiety or panic symptoms.

DIAGNOSIS: ACCENTUATE THE PEARLS, AVOID THE POTHOLES

Not all depressive moods and syndromes are the same. There are diagnostic potholes to be aware of and navigate around to improve the likelihood of resolution of the symptoms and optimize functioning. It is not enough to notice that a patient with cancer feels depressed or even has a history of depression. The causes of depressive symptoms are many and varied. The mental health professional will note the patient's psychiatric history, family history of depression, current stressors, current medications or treatments that can cause depression, current comorbidities that can bring on depressive or demoralization symptoms, as well as the time course and context of the onset and occurrence of the symptoms. Depressive moods or symptoms do not necessarily add up to a definitive reason to treat with a medication. However, suspicions that your patient has a more serious depressive episode, rather than transient sad or depressive feelings as a reaction to having a cancer diagnosis, a recurrence of cancer, or going through cancer treatment, are strengthened by the presence of risk factors. Risk factors for depressive syndromes in cancer patients and how this syndrome looks symptomatically are highlighted in Boxes 1.1 and 1.2.

ALGORITHM FOR DIAGNOSING A SYNDROME OF DEPRESSION IN CANCER PATIENTS

Depressed mood and anhedonia (a significant loss of interest or ability to experience pleasure in activities they used to enjoy), while considering other circumstances such as life or medical stressors or losses, including pain that is not well controlled, fatigue, urinary or bowel incontinence, recent retirement, or the death of loved ones, that make activity difficult or less enjoyable rather than the symptoms of depression being the culprit.

+

Risk factors: personal or family history of depression; advanced disease; pancreatic, head and neck, or lung cancer; substance use, substance abuse or intoxication, substance cessation, substance withdrawal; history of suicide attempt

+

Cognitive aspects of depression severity: hopelessness + worthlessness or guilt and feeling like a burden + suicidal ideation, or ruminating thoughts of wanting to die

+

Consideration of *neurovegetative symptoms* such as loss of appetite, fatigue, clouded concentration, or change in sleep habits and the degree to which these symptoms may be due to complications of the cancer or cancer treatment rather than the development of a major depressive syndrome. This may take detective collaboration with the oncology team:

If physical symptoms are correlated with a patient's demoralization and frustration and lack of engagement in or enjoyment of activities, ask the patient the following:
"If you could get a pill to make your energy, sleep, appetite, or pain better, what would you want to do?"
The person *without* a major depression might tell you the activities that he or she would love to engage in, now and in the future.

> The depressed patient might easily shrug her shoulders and say, "It doesn't matter; I don't care."

=

Depressive syndrome that may respond to an antidepressant

Sometimes depressive syndromes can be accompanied by other symptoms that may not resolve from an antidepressant alone. Because it can take 4–8 weeks for an antidepressant to resolve depressive symptoms, it can be frustrating to wait 2 months without any relief, and can inadvertently add to a patient's suffering. The following uncomfortable symptoms, which may be part of or exist concurrently with a depressive disorder, are important to identify and address before an antidepressant has time to be effective:

Box 1.1 RISK FACTORS FOR DEPRESSIVE SYNDROMES IN CANCER PATIENTS

- Previous history of depression (and/or anxiety) disorder
- Patient has more advanced cancer
- Pancreatic, lung, and head and neck cancers
- Patient has poorly controlled pain
- Patient has had other life stresses or recent losses
- Social isolation
- Recent history of substance use or cessation of alcohol or tobacco use
- Hopelessness
- Worthlessness and guilt
- Suicidal ideation

- Restlessness (an anxiolytic might help)
- Insomnia (an anxiolytic, atypical antipsychotic, or hypnotic may help)
- Irritability (an anxiolytic or atypical antipsychotic may be helpful)
- Nausea (an antiemetic, some antipsychotics, or benzodiazepines might help)
- Pain or other physical discomforts: address those symptoms in addition to treating the depression

---

Box 1.2 ISOLATED SYMPTOMS IN CANCER PATIENTS
THAT MAY LOOK LIKE DEPRESSION BUT DO NOT NECESSARILY
MAKE A DISORDER

- Sadness
- Demoralization
- Anger or irritability
- Fatigue
- Thoughts about death

MEDICAL LOOK-A-LIKES

Metabolic, nutritional, and endocrine disorders such as abnormal levels of potassium, sodium, or calcium, deficiencies of folate or vitamin B_{12}, hypothyroidism, hyperthyroidism, or adrenal insufficiency can produce depressive symptoms (Box 1.3), as can cognitive deficits, fatigue, pain, and substance use, thus further complicating practitioners' consideration of a diagnosis of major depression. A

Box 1.3 LOOK-A-LIKE EXPLANATIONS OF DEPRESSIVE SYMPTOMS

- Cognitive disorder—chemo-brain or hormone brain (a spectrum of concentration deficits caused by chemotherapy or hormonal treatment for cancer, in one or more of the following skills: attention, memory, multitasking, and planning and organizing abilities).
- Fatigue—complaints of physical depletion that may be related to cancer treatment or the cancer or depression; however, a solitary fatigue symptom with subsequent decreased activity or social engagement can be mistaken for a depressive episode.
- Inadequately treated pain—pain is a subjectively measured symptom that can lead to depression if not adequately treated, but it can also be mistaken for depression if the subjective complaints exceed what is considered the norm, and the patient does not engage in usually pleasurable activities.
- Other medical disorders or electrolyte or vitamin abnormalities
  - Thyroid function abnormalities
  - Vitamin B_{12} deficiency
  - Folate deficiency
  - Metabolic abnormalities
    - Hypercalcemia
    - Sodium, potassium imbalance
    - Anemia
  - Alcohol and substance abuse
  - Infectious disease
  - Hyper- or hypocortisolemia
  - Cognitive impairment

primary care doctor, nurse practitioner, physician assistant, or on-cologist can order laboratory tests for abnormalities that can cause depressive symptoms.

Said the non-prescriber to the prescriber: "Are there other pos-sible causes of these depressive symptoms to consider that might change the treatment plan?"

The correct answer is "Of course." It never hurts to consider a dif-ferential diagnosis (potential alternative diagnostic considerations given the combination of presenting symptoms and variables).

KEY FACTORS TO CONSIDER WHEN DIAGNOSING DEPRESSION

The intensity of depressive symptoms as well as their persistence may help define a clinical syndrome. The time course of the appearance, continuation, and fluctuation of a depressive syndrome can be im-portant in deciding whether an antidepressant might be indicated. A first responder clinician might ask if the symptoms are present most days and for most of each day. How long have the symptoms been there? A 2-week time frame is a primary benchmark for identifying a major depression. Are the symptoms worse at any part of the day or evening? Do the feelings coincide with physical symptoms, such as pain, nausea, vomiting, or gastric distress such as constipation or diarrhea? Does the patient experience cognitive slowing? Does the timeline of symptoms coincide with the beginning or completion of a medication regimen for the cancer or another disorder? Cognitive slowing can be related to depression but can also be a current or af-tereffect complication of chemotherapy or other treatment.

ASK, BECAUSE THEY MAY NOT TELL

Even if you are not prescribing any medication, you should ask the patient what medications and supplements they are taking. Sometimes these details get lost in brief prescriber visits or with patients' decreased disclosure of medications that they do not think are "important," even with the recent emphasis in hospitals and ambulatory clinics on asking for home medication reconciliation lists. Ask! And ask for updates periodically. Suggest that patients write down their medications and give the list to each prescriber they visit. You may find, for instance, that the recent addition of a supplement has caused lethargy that is leading to depressive symptoms, or restlessness that manifests as anxiety or insomnia.

The following questions may aid clinicians in considering an antidepressant medication:

- Are the symptoms ongoing or sporadic?
  - Ongoing symptoms more likely require an antidepressant.
- Is the depressed mood and loss of pleasure in life activities ongoing for the majority of the day, for most days of the week, for at least 2 weeks?
  - These are the classic gateway symptoms of depression that often warrant an antidepressant, assuming the symptoms cannot be temporally explained by the cancer or treatment or another medical disorder.
- Are the symptoms situation specific or stressor specific, or are they free-floating or generalized?

- Free-floating or generalized symptoms more likely require an antidepressant.
- Are the symptoms a recurrence of a previous disorder?
  - If yes, this is a potentially significant indicator for an antidepressant.
- Are the symptoms new since the cancer diagnosis or a cancer recurrence, or since notification of no further available cancer treatment?
  - Severity of current depressive symptoms may indicate benefit of an antidepressant.
- Are the depressive symptoms due to a medical cause or aberration?
  - An antidepressant may not help. Can the medical abnormality be corrected?
- Are neurovegetative (NV) symptoms (e.g., changes in sleep, appetite, weight, concentration, and energy levels) in the context of profound depression caused by the cancer or cancer treatment? The timing of the onset of these NV symptoms while taking into consideration potential medical triggers and ongoing depressive symptoms for at least 2 weeks most of the day, most days, may be helpful clues to indicate the benefits of an antidepressant, while possibly fixing the medical issues at the same time.
  - If a patient is not having a major depressive episode, an antidepressant might be able to target one or more NV symptoms to aid sleep (e.g., a sedating antidepressant), appetite (e.g., mirtazapine or other antidepressants that can cause weight gain), or energy (e.g., bupropion). If the symptoms correlate with a major depression, traditional dosing of an antidepressant is warranted.
  - If addressing individual symptoms of fatigue, pain, or gastric upset does not resolve the depressed mood, an antidepressant is warranted.

- If the patient is older than age 70 years or frail, are somatic complaints of malaise or achiness more reflective of a depressive disorder than of aging or a medical condition?
  - Again, the timing of onset and continuity of symptoms will guide a prescriber. If the prescriber sees a chronic level of malaise and achiness that was not previously correlated with depression, or sees these symptoms set in with a depressed mood and anhedonia, an antidepressant is likely to be prescribed.
- Are the depressive symptoms due to recent lifestyle changes such as substance, tobacco, or alcohol cessation because of the cancer diagnosis?
  - Make sure to monitor for withdrawal symptoms and advocate for addressing those symptoms with safer replacement medications and substance-specific abstinence coping therapy to replace the substance that in the past helped the patient cope with stress but in unhealthy ways.
- One of the most important gauges for whether an antidepressant would be helpful is whether the depressive symptoms are appreciably interfering with the patient's ability to carry on and enjoy life, even with cancer.
- Does the patient have difficulty engaging in behavioral interventions (physical or occupational therapy, writing or art therapy, etc.) because they have fallen into an all-or-nothing syndrome that may be related to depression ("nothing is worthwhile, and nothing can help")?
  - Communication among all caregivers is important. If the patient is deemed capable of participating in occupational or physical therapy or can be active behaviorally but does not show the motivation to attend or participate, and there is not a good medical (or another psychiatric) explanation,

in the setting of other depressive symptoms, an antidepressant may be warranted.

Regardless of whether an antidepressant or supplemental medication is suggested by prescribers, ongoing support by non-prescribing clinicians is vital.

DEPRESSION CASES

Throughout this book, we present a few fictionalized clinical scenarios, or cases. In this chapter, we follow Joanne, Jake, and John through the diagnostic and treatment phases of their depressive syndromes. We point out the pearls and potholes to be aware of diagnostically and therapeutically, and toward the end of the chapter, we discuss the medication suggestions that we would hope would bring relief.

INTRODUCING: JOANNE

Joanne is a 77-year-old widowed woman. She is a retired music critic. She loves classical music and Mozart in particular. Joanne was diagnosed with breast cancer about a year ago and had a mastectomy with subsequent chemotherapy and has been on tamoxifen for the past 6 months. "I wonder when the other shoe will fall. My mother died of breast cancer when it returned all over her body 6 years after her treatment."

She has been receiving supportive therapy from a local therapist for the past 3 months to address her fears of recurrence and for "just not feeling like myself." She complains to her therapist of

---

weakness and fatigue that have worsened during the past few weeks. She stopped reading the newspaper and has noticed some trouble multitasking and feeling more forgetful. "I don't feel as sharp as I used to." She no longer feels like taking her daily walk in the local park, which she used to do religiously. Although she is tired and naps during the day, she has difficulty falling asleep and staying asleep. She has little appetite and does not want to eat regularly, and she eventually tells her therapist, "This is not what I signed up for." Occasionally, she feels like she does not want to live in a weakened state; however, she adamantly states that she does not want to hurt herself. She is easily tearful and says she feels depressed most of the day for most days of the week.

She still listens to Mozart at home and writes a weekly music blog, but she has found it more difficult and less pleasurable during the past few weeks. She has stopped going to concerts.

Key Factors in Joanne's Depressive Picture

Fear of cancer recurrence	*Worry/anxiety*
Does not feel as sharp as she used to	*Cognitive slowing*
Increasingly depressed and tearful	*Depressed mood*
Fatigue and decreased sleep	*Fatigue and insomnia*
Stopped going to concerts	*Social isolation*
Decreased appetite	*Appetite*
Finds less pleasure in activities	*Anhedonia*
Doesn't want to live like this	*Thoughts of dying*
Duration of symptoms	*More than 2 weeks*

INTRODUCING: JAKE

Jake is a 58-year-old man never smoker who was diagnosed with metastatic lung cancer approximately 3 years ago. He has been treated with radiation and chemotherapy. He had high hopes when he started an experimental trial of a new immune checkpoint inhibitor, a programmed cell death (PD-1) immunotherapy medication; however, he found out a few weeks ago that his cancer was not responding to this medication and the cancer was spreading quickly. He is in your oncology clinic for a discussion of another clinical trial for a phase 1 medication, which he is a good candidate for because his energy and appetite have remained unchanged and his performance level has been adequate for the trial. Jake's wife tells you, the clinic nurse, that his mood has been down most of the day, most days of the week, since finding out about the progression of his disease. He has become more hopeless, feeling he will not live to the same age as his father, who died at age 70 years of a heart attack. He has become more socially withdrawn and does not even enjoy spending time with his children or friends. He says he is not sure if it matters whether he lives or dies anymore, as he would like to avoid the suffering that will surely come as his body deteriorates from his cancer. He also adamantly states he will not hurt himself because he knows how painful that could be for his family. He says, "I do not want another medication to raise my hopes, just to have it not work, and that might only cause more suffering."

Jake meets criteria for a major depression. His primary symptoms of depression include depressed mood for more than 2 weeks, anhedonia, hopelessness, and social withdrawal. He is too depressed even to consider going on the clinical trial. Given his metastatic lung cancer, the primary oncology team will check to determine if there are any chemistry abnormalities (i.e., hypercalcemia and hyponatremia) as well as other medical anomalies (i.e., hypoxia and hypothyroidism) that could otherwise explain his depressive symptomatology. They assessed that he has no active suicidal ideation or intent or plan to hurt himself. While they are waiting for the laboratory test results, they agree with Jake and his wife that treatment for depression should start immediately.

TREATMENT CONSIDERATIONS

Important Information to Know About Antidepressant Meds for Heads

If the symptoms of depression continue to interfere with enjoyment in living, once other medical causes are ruled out or alleviated as best as possible, it makes sense to start an antidepressant. Patients can be told about numerous studies cited in the Institute of Medicine's 2008 report[2] on the effectiveness of antidepressant medications in cancer patients.

Once a prescriber decides to treat major depression with an antidepressant, the non-prescriber should continue supportive therapy that likely includes cognitive behaviorally oriented therapy components to realistically reframe negative thought processes and encourage physical activity such as walking. The prescribing psycho-oncology clinician would consider all symptoms that may be addressable under the umbrella of depression. The combination of psychotropic medication and psychotherapy is the most effective method to treat depression. Other modalities may help as well. For instance, exercise can be one of the most effective ways for improving cancer-related fatigue. If aerobic exercise and strength training are done regularly, they may also have similar results as an antidepressant for mild to moderate depression. So even prescribing clinicians may not make a medication their first recommendation, although the standard of care for moderate to severe depression is often a combination of medication and nonmedication recommendations, including psychotherapy, exercise, meditation, and making lifestyle changes as appropriate.

GETTING TO KNOW THE ANTIDEPRESSANTS

Non-prescribing clinicians should become familiar with the psychotropic medications their patients are on. Box 1.4 lists the most commonly used antidepressants to treat depression in cancer patients. The brand names and generic names of the newer antidepressants as well as the older, less commonly used medications are listed so that readers can start to become better acquainted with the medications. Many are described in greater detail in this chapter. These medications include the selective serotonin reuptake inhibitors (SSRIs), the serotonin norepinephrine reuptake inhibitors (SNRIs), other antidepressants, as well as psychostimulants,

Box 1.4 COMMONLY PRESCRIBED MEDICATIONS TO TREAT
DEPRESSIVE SYNDROMES

Drug Class, Generic Name, and Brand Name
SSRIS

Citalopram (Celexa)

Escitalopram (Lexapro)

Fluoxetine (Prozac)

Paroxetine (Paxil)

Sertraline (Zoloft)

Vilazodone (Viibryd)

SNRIS

Venlafaxine (Effexor)

Desvenlafaxine (Pristiq)

Duloxetine (Cymbalta)

Milnacipran (Ixel, Savella, Dalcipran, Toledomin)

OTHER ANTIDEPRESSANTS

Mirtazapine (Remeron)—primarily works on serotonin, as
well as norepinephrine and histamine

Bupropion (Wellbutrin)—primarily works on dopamine
and norepinephrine

Vortioxetine (Trintellix)—considered a serotonin mod-
ulator, and not SSRI specifically, because it works
on multiple locations of neuron, synapse, and
transporters

TRICYCLIC ANTIDEPRESSANTS (OLDER, LESS COMMONLY USED
ANTIDEPRESSANTS)

Amitriptyline (Elavil)—primarily works on serotonin and
norepinephrine

Imipramine (Tofranil)—primarily works on serotonin and
norepinephrine

Nortriptyline (Pamelor)—metabolite of amitriptyline; primarily works on serotonin and norepinephrine

Desipramine (Norpramin)—metabolite of imipramine; primarily works on norepinephrine and serotonin

Doxepin (Sinequan)—primarily works on serotonin, norepinephrine, and histamine; used for sleep and to ease
pruritis (severe itching of the skin)

Trazodone (Desyrel)—heterocyclic antidepressant; primarily works on serotonin; used more often as a sedating
agent for insomnia

MONOAMINE OXIDASE INHIBITORS (OLDER AND RARELY USED IN
THE CANCER SETTING)

These medications block the activity of monoamine oxidase enzymes, which is another mechanism for preventing
presynaptic neuronal reuptake in order to maintain norepinephrine, serotonin, and dopamine in the synapse.

Phenelzine (Nardil)
Tranylcypromine (Parnate)
Isocarboxazid (Marplan)

WAKEFULNESS AGENTS

These agents have an unclear mechanism of action; they may work on dopamine, histamine, norepinephrine, serotonin, orexin, or glutamate systems.

Modafinil (Provigil)
Armodafinil (Nuvigil)

PSYCHOSTIMULANTS

These likely work on dopamine, norepinephrine, and serotonin transmitters.

Methylphenidate (Ritalin, Concerta, Metadate)
Dexmethylphenidate (Focalin)
Dextroamphetamine (Dexedrine)
Mixed amphetamine salts (Adderall)

tricyclic antidepressants (TCAs), and monoamine oxidase inhibitors (MAOIs). The advantages and disadvantages of these medications in various oncology situations are described later in the chapter so non-prescribers can be even better educated advocates for their patients. "Off-label" uses of the antidepressants, such as reducing hot flashes, alleviating neuropathic pain, stimulating appetite, decreasing nausea, lifting fatigue, and improving sleep, are also discussed. The antidepressants primarily exert their benefits by modulating the following brain neurotransmitters dopamine, serotonin, and/or norepinephrine.

How Antidepressants Work and Why It Is Good for the Non-Prescriber and Patients to Know

Non-psychiatric prescribers dispense most antidepressant prescriptions written in the United States. Most of these prescriptions come from primary care physicians (PCPs). In the cancer setting, oncologists likely prescribe a majority of these medications for their patients when psychiatrists or PCPs are not readily available or when visits with psychiatrists are not covered well enough by health insurance, so patients would otherwise go without adequate treatment for their depression. Patients are more adherent to taking antidepressants, as with all other medications, when they understand how to take them properly and know what to watch for. Many patients do not fill antidepressant prescriptions even when they are given—sometimes because they are skittish about taking one more medication, sometimes because they are ambivalent about acknowledging a psychiatric disorder or concerned about possible side effects, and sometimes because they do not fully understand how their depression may get in the way of their cancer treatment.

Approximately 10% of adults in the United States fill one or more antidepressant prescriptions each year.[3] Many people who start taking an antidepressant for 1 month will not take it for the second month; in fact, most people wind up taking the medication for less than 3 months, although it is usually recommended that patients take the antidepressant for 9–12 months after it starts working. The reasons for this variability in following through with prescription recommendations range from not understanding clearly what to do, to having uncomfortable side effects, to not having sufficient follow-up with their prescriber, or having misinformation about the medication (Box 1.5). Sometimes patients are given samples of new

---

Box 1.5 MYTHS THAT KEEP PATIENTS FROM TAKING
ANTIDEPRESSANTS

"I don't need to take it every day."

"I don't want to get addicted."

"I can stop it once I start feeling better."

"If it hasn't started working in a couple of weeks, it won't
work at all."

"All antidepressants are the same; if one doesn't work well,
none will."

"My friend took an antidepressant [or any prescribed medi-
cation] and had a bad reaction; I don't want that."

"Since medications are expensive, I can make them last twice
as long if I break them in half."

"Antidepressants change the essence of who you are."

"Over-the-counter stress relievers and supplements are just as
good as prescription medications, and they are safer too."

---

expensive antidepressants that may not be covered by their insurance company or will require expensive copayments that the patient
cannot afford. So, they stop taking the medication. Thus, an important role of the non-prescriber (as well as the prescriber) is to ask if,
how, and when the patient is taking the medication. If it isn't taken
regularly, it won't work.

Antidepressants are taken by mouth and absorbed from the stomach into the bloodstream. They are distributed throughout the body

and eventually to the brain for their onset of action. They primarily get metabolized and broken down in the liver and eventually get excreted. Genetic differences in a small percentage of patients and interactions with other medications can slow down or speed up metabolism in the liver, leading to less or more availability of the medication to do its job; in slow metabolizers, there is the possibility of having too much medication available and the development of toxic side effects. Those with compromised kidney function may be at risk of electrolyte abnormalities. You don't have to be a neuroscientist to get the gist of how these medications work, but getting the gist, and passing it along to your patients, may be among the most important guidance that increases openness to considering an antidepressant treatment, as well as improving reliability in following proper instructions and therefore improving the likely outcome. When Dr. Roth considers prescribing an antidepressant, he draws the schematic illustrations shown in figures 1.1–1.5 on pages 22–26 in his office for his patients.

Disclaimer: The neural circuitry of depression and how antidepressants work are extremely complex and still being elucidated. Multiple areas of the brain and many neuropsychiatric variables are in play to cause biological changes needed to relieve depression. The figures shown in this chapter are drastically streamlined and schematized to illustrate one feature of a complex, multifaceted process. Please do not think that these even approach exact replicas of the very intricate and interconnected pathways in our brains. But these schematics can be drawn while the patient is in the office and may improve a person's appreciation of why the medication will not work instantaneously (as a minor tranquilizer might) and why the medication needs to be taken daily for at least a few weeks before it is likely to start working. When people get a better grasp of how a medication is functioning in their body, they feel more engaged in the process. And for those patients who like to

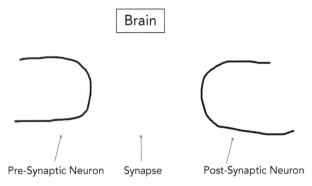

Figure 1.1. Two neurons (nerve cells) in a brain separated by a synapse.

use visualization techniques in their engagement with a therapy, this may be a constructive set of images.

The brain is made of many neurons (cells) with many different functions. Figure 1.1 shows two neurons separated by a synapse (a space). The neuron to the left of the space is considered the presynaptic neuron, and the one on the right is the postsynaptic neuron. In this figure, the chemical action, or direction of traffic, goes from left to right, with chemicals (called neurotransmitters) flowing from the presynaptic neuron, through the synapse, to the postsynaptic neuron.

DR. ROTH'S NITTY-GRITTY REPRESENTATION OF THE BRAIN (A SKY VIEW OF THE BRAIN AND HOW ANTIDEPRESSANTS WORK)

Chemicals in the brain called neurotransmitters are made in cells called neurons (presynaptic) as an early step in the process to prevent significant depression or anxiety. These neurotransmitters are excreted from the presynaptic neuron into an adjacent space (synapse), where they then travel to make contact with a specially matched receptor on a (postsynaptic) neuron on the other side of the synapse. The neurotransmitters that generally regulate mood and anxiety symptoms are serotonin, norepinephrine, and dopamine (Figure 1.2).

But just because the neurotransmitters are manufactured in the presynaptic neuron does not mean a person cannot get depressed or anxious. The serotonin, norepinephrine, and dopamine transmitters are shipped out of the presynaptic neuron into a space called a synapse, in search of an adjacent postsynaptic neuron upon which to make contact.

It is still not possible to determine if a patient's depression is more serotonin, norepinephrine, or dopamine based and what mechanism in its functioning has gone awry; a test that could identify these could make medication choices more accurate. There are new tests that may indicate whether a patient's genetic structure will make them able to appropriately metabolize and tolerate a specific antidepressant in the liver P450 protein processing metabolism system. These tests may indicate if a patient will be responsive to the active antidepressant effect, and not have critical side effects, or toxicity. Unfortunately, the genetic tests are in their scientific

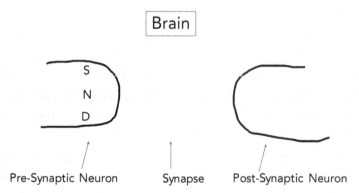

Figure 1.2. The serotonin, norepinephrine, and dopamine neurotransmitters in the brain regulate mood and anxiety symptoms. S, serotonin; N, norepinephrine; D, dopamine.

infancy, they are expensive, they are not always covered by insurance, and they cannot yet indicate whether one antidepressant is chemically appropriate to treat any individual's neurodepressive syndrome; these tests only measure whether abnormal metabolism will interfere with a potential response. Currently, it does not appear to be worth trading clinical experience for most routine depressive episodes with an expensive genetic test. This technology may be helpful if a patient does not respond to first- or second-line treatment, has treatment-limiting side effects, or if they or a family member has previously had trouble tolerating antidepressants.

A CLOSE-UP VIEW OF THE BRAIN

A Presynaptic Neuron and the Neurotransmitters It Produces

Once the transmitter is released into the synapse, it searches for its matching contact points on the adjacent neuron. This is often described as a key (neurotransmitter) and lock (receptor) fit.

Ideally, when a neurotransmitter (key) is released from the presynaptic neuron into the synapse it will identify and connect with a matching receptor (lock): serotonin transmitter with a serotonin receptor, norepinephrine transmitter with a norepinephrine receptor, or dopamine transmitter with a dopamine receptor. Adequate linking of neurotransmitters (keys) and receptors (locks) improves the excitation efficiency and functioning of the mood regulatory system (Figure 1.3).

Our examples now focus on SSRIs in order to simplify the discussion, although the process is similar for norepinephrine and dopamine reuptake inhibition as well.

There is still much to be learned about the biological causes of severe depression and anxiety. Hypotheses include that chronic stress

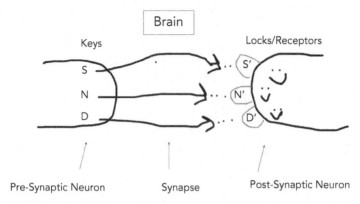

Figure 1.3. Adequate linking of neurotransmitters (keys) and receptors (locks) improves the excitation efficiency and functioning of the mood regulatory system. S, serotonin; N, norepinephrine; D, dopamine.

exposure can lead to decreased synaptic density or a suboptimal supply of viable and properly working receptors on the postsynaptic neuron. When unused serotonin accumulates in the synapse, a homeostatic mechanism kicks in because the environment does not like unusable material amassing, so transmitters that do not link with a receptor are metabolized, or taken back (reuptake), into the original presynaptic neuron and broken down (Figure 1.4).

Along comes an antidepressant that is a reuptake inhibitor. This reuptake inhibitor prevents the serotonin from being taken back into the presynaptic neuron from the synapse to get metabolized and recycled. When an SSRI antidepressant blocks serotonin from going back in, the synapse starts to flood with serotonin. Newer serotonergic-oriented antidepressants (mirtazapine, vortioxetine, and vilazodone) have additional actions that may relieve other symptoms of depression, such as anxiety, insomnia, and gastric upset. Similarly, an SNRI (venlafaxine, desvenlafaxine, duloxetine, or levomilnacipran) will prevent serotonin and norepinephrine from leaving the synapse, making more serotonin

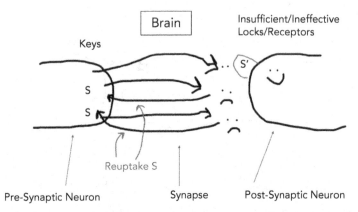

Figure 1.4. Transmitters that do not link with a receptor are metabolized, or taken back (reuptake), into the original presynaptic neuron and broken down. S, serotonin.

and norepinephrine neurotransmitters available to postsynaptic receptors. The reuptake inhibition in effect builds a wall that does not allow the neurotransmitters to exit the synapse and re-enter the presynaptic neuron. This process occurs within days of starting the antidepressant (Figure 1.5).

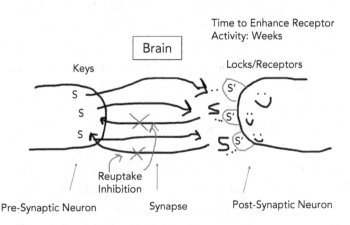

Figure 1.5. Medications that block reuptake prevent the neurotransmitters from re-entering the presynaptic neuron. They stay in the synapse. S, serotonin.

BUT THE THERAPEUTIC EFFECTS DO NOT BEGIN FOR AT LEAST 2 WEEKS AND MAYBE NOT EVEN FOR 5 OR 6 WEEKS

Why?

It is not just the quantity of serotonin, norepinephrine, or dopamine transmitters that improves mood or anxiety. As the neurotransmitters are continually seen in abundance in the synapse, the postsynaptic neuron and its receptors essentially morph and get recharged. So, with an SSRI medication, the postsynaptic neuron basically says, "Hey, look at all that available serotonin. Let's get some better transmission going!" Again, there are many minute variables involved in this very complicated process, some of which are still unknown.

During the next few weeks, and sometimes for up to 6 weeks or longer, receptors and the transmitter–receptor connections become more plentiful and efficient, hopefully leading to improved mood and anxiety.

This same complex process also happens when an SNRI leads to enhanced serotonin and norepinephrine transmission or when a dopamine reuptake inhibitor (DRI) is used to enrich dopaminergic synaptic conduction. Most important, this is not an instantaneous process—it takes time for the postsynaptic receptors to improve their connectivity.

HOW PSYCHO-ONCOLOGY PRESCRIBERS CHOOSE AN ANTIDEPRESSANT AND MAXIMIZE THE BENEFITS OF ANTIDEPRESSANT TREATMENT (AND HOW A NON-PRESCRIBER FITS IN)

The Short List of Benefits of Antidepressants

The list of side effects in medication package inserts for any medication is usually far longer than the list of benefits. The official list of benefits for antidepressants will indicate the medication is for the treatment of several conditions not limited to major depressive disorder, including generalized anxiety disorder, obsessive–compulsive disorder, and panic disorder. Other uses are not always included in original indications but are found to have benefits anecdotally or in small studies, some of which are considered off-label benefits that can be helpful for people with cancer or the medically ill in general. Some antidepressants can aid in the treatment of hot flashes (for menopausal women or men with prostate cancer on androgen deprivation therapy), neuropathic pain syndromes, loss of appetite, nausea, and sleep disturbance.

Given the routine mechanisms of action diagrammed previously, it is not clear why some antidepressants work to relieve depression in some patients and not others, why some people tolerate one medication but not another, or why some people have problematic drug interactions with other medications and other people do not.

Patients may metabolize medications at different speeds because of genetic presence or absence of metabolizing enzymes in their liver or because of competition for access to metabolizing enzymes based on other medications or medical problems. The major system for metabolizing medications in the liver is called the P450 system. Many tables exist to highlight potential drug–drug interactions that will either enhance or slow down (inhibit) metabolism of a medication. We will not go into detail about these medications or potential interactions. That they may occur is important for the prescriber to know. However, it can be helpful for patients to understand why medications do not act the same for all patients.

Just because one medication does not work for a patient does not mean that another medication, even in the same class (SSRI or SNRI), will not work. But the usual treatment strategy after an antidepressant does not work after a thorough trial (at least 6 weeks at each therapeutic dose increase, with dose increases as appropriate) is to try a medication from a different class of antidepressants. Therefore, if an SSRI did not work, the next choice of antidepressant might be to switch to an SNRI or add an adjunct dose of bupropion or low dose of mirtazapine, which can improve the efficacy of the SSRI. It is important to identify and treat ancillary symptoms such as insomnia, anxiety, nausea, or pain, which may impede more complete improvement. In these prolonged response situations, the non-prescriber may be in the best position to encourage a patient to continue treatment and maintain hope with support to continue adjuvant psychotherapy. Reminders to patients that incomplete treatment may be a harbinger of poorer functioning in the future may help them stay the course. Early discontinuation of antidepressant treatment, or incomplete remission of the depression, increases the likelihood of relapse. Updates from a non-prescriber about whether side effects from the antidepressant (e.g., fatigue or unexpected anxiety) are interfering with the potential benefits of the medication may help a prescriber fine-tune the antidepressant treatment.

Almost all antidepressants have similar efficacy for treating a major depression. They generally take 2 to 5 or 6 weeks to kick in at any one dose if they are going to work at all. Again, it is still not clear why some patients will respond to one antidepressant and other patients may not. If patients do not realize it could take weeks to feel the benefits, they may stop the medication prematurely. That is not a failure of the medication but of a suboptimal communication process or inadequate understanding. If a patient had a good response to an antidepressant in the past, that antidepressant is often a good medication to start now, assuming there is no current contraindication to using that medication in the cancer context. However, a patient who responded to an old-line antidepressant in her 30s may not tolerate the same medication in her 70s because of current medical problems, side effects, or potentially conflicting medications.

One of the more common side effects of these medications is an energizing effect, which may be helpful if the person has fatigue. Bupropion is likely to have an energizing effect and is sometimes used when patients complain of fatigue. But if the energizing effect overshoots, it may be experienced as anxiety or restlessness, and it can lead to insomnia if it occurs at night. Irritability, short-temperedness, and increased argumentativeness can also be associated with this hyperarousal or hyperreactive side effect.

Alternatively, some antidepressants can cause a calming effect, which is not bad for those who are feeling stressed. Too much of this effect, however, results in grogginess. If someone became more fatigued from an antidepressant, we might first recommend taking the medication at nighttime because it may induce better nighttime sleep. But if a patient already has daytime fatigue that has now worsened, this side effect could be a deal breaker. The antidepressants most likely to have a calming effect include the TCAs, citalopram, and mirtazapine. They may work well for those having trouble falling asleep. Trazodone and doxepin are sedating antidepressants that in low doses are more often used for inducing sleep than for treating depression, as the higher doses needed to treat depression lead to too much daytime sedation and cognitive cloudiness.

Some depressive syndromes may improve on their own, but if the suffering of depression can be lessened more quickly by a medication, and a patient's functioning and safety can be improved, then why not maximize the medication's efficacy and limit the drawbacks? A majority of people with depressive syndromes will have some response to initial antidepressant therapy, whereas fewer will have a full remission. This leaves a significant number of people who may respond to a modification of the treatment approach, with adjustment of dosing or adding or changing medications by a practitioner who is practiced and comfortable with psychotropic medications. So, it pays to try one, and then try another if needed, if the symptoms are significant and ongoing. Primary prescribers may also refer to psychiatric experts if needed.

It is important to note that neurovegetative symptoms often are the earliest to improve with antidepressant treatment. A patient who has improvement in sleep and energy and is starting to enjoy some activities, but whose mood remains depressed at first, should be encouraged by all providers to stay the course. The mood often improves last.

Making Antidepressants Multitask: The Benefits May Offer Twofers

Although we want to reduce the harmful or uncomfortable side effects of medications, sometimes with medically ill populations, antidepressants may have a beneficial secondary side effect profile that addresses a specific symptom (e.g., fatigue, insomnia, or weight loss) so the prescriber (and patient) can get a "twofer" with one medication (Table 1.1). Each of the questions listed in

Table 1.1 A Sky View of Antidepressant Multitasking
Twofers—Positive Secondary Effects

Patient Is Depressed And	Prescriber Can Consider
Has decreased appetite	Mirtazapine, TCA, psychostimulant
Has gastric upset or nausea	Mirtazapine
Has fatigue	Psychostimulant, bupropion
Has difficulty falling asleep or staying asleep	Mirtazapine, trazodone
Has anxiety	Mirtazapine, SSRI
Has neuropathic pain	Duloxetine, milnacipran, some SSRIs
Is on tamoxifen	Venlafaxine, desvenlafaxine, citalopram, escitalopram, mirtazapine
Is nearing the end of life	Psychostimulant

SSRI, selective serotonin reuptake inhibitor; TCA, tricyclic antidepressant.

Box 1.6 might lead to a branching decision-tree investigation to determine if and how the problematic symptom can be remedied. The same box is presented later in the chapter with recommended solutions after we review the medications in more detail. If the symptom is secondary to depression, both the symptom and the depression would be treated simultaneously with an antidepressant. Some bothersome symptoms that may be part of depression, such as insomnia, fatigue, anxiety, or loss of appetite, may be helped concurrently by a medication in another class, such

Box 1.6 QUESTIONS TO HELP DETECT MULTIPLE BENEFITS
FOR AN ANTIDEPRESSANT[A]

Is the patient having trouble with asleep?

If yes, does the patient get to sleep fine but wakes up
often in the middle of the night?

If they do, is it because they have other physical
symptoms, such as pain, urinary frequency,
gastric upset, or cough? These symptoms need
to be addressed medically if possible. Sedating
someone sufficiently to sleep through a physical
issue can be helpful, but could also lead to a wet
bed or one full of feces in the morning or, rarely,
an aspiration pneumonia (a lung infection that
develops if food, liquid, or vomit is inhaled, that
may occur more easily when a person is lying flat
and coughing).

Can consider sedating antidepressants or an atypical
antipsychotic.

Does the patient get back to sleep within 20–30 minutes
of awakening?

If yes, no medication is needed. May try relaxation or imaging techniques and reviewing sleep
hygiene.

Is the patient eating well?

Is there no or low appetite, or a decrease or change in
taste?

Consider an appetite stimulant or an antidepressant.

Does the patient have a neuropathic pain syndrome?

Consider an SSRI or a TCA.

Does the patient have daytime fatigue or trouble staying awake?

Consider a stimulating medication.

Is the patient having difficulty with concentrating?

Consider neurocognitive testing or brain imaging to ensure there is no medical cause from cancer or cancer treatment (i.e., chemotherapy, radiation therapy, or opioids).

Consider a stimulating medication.

Does the patient have hot flashes that awaken them frequently at night?

Consider a medication that addresses hot flashes.

Is the patient feeling anxious?

Consider an antidepressant or short-term benzodiazepine.

ªSpecific solutions noted in Box 1.13 on pages 64, 65.

as a hypnotic, benzodiazepine, psychostimulant, or an atypical antipsychotic, until the antidepressant has had a chance to be effective (at least 2 weeks) (Figure 1.6). In addition, poor appetite, gastric problems, fatigue, and pain can all be treated with noninvasive suggestions such as serving smaller portions of food, changing diet, meditation, behavioral activation, and physical or occupational therapy.

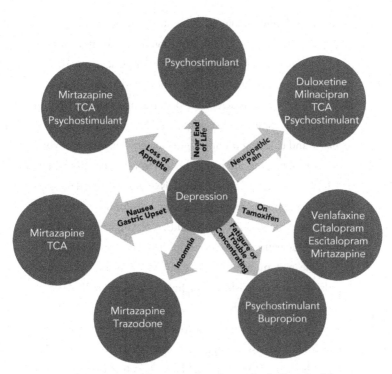

Figure 1.6. Choosing an antidepressant based on individual medical factors.

INTRODUCING: JOHN

John is a 64-year-old recently retired man with metastatic prostate cancer who has been on the androgen deprivation therapy (ADT) agent leuprolide for a few years; docetaxel chemotherapy was added a few months ago for progression of his disease. His only other medical issue is hypertension, for which he is on hydrochlorothiazide (a diuretic). He started seeing a psychotherapist to help deal with his fear of becoming debilitated and dependent on his wife, who struggles with multiple sclerosis. He was initially given a diagnosis of adjustment disorder with depressed mood. He feels tired much of the day. The behavioral activation the therapist recommended was going well and John was walking regularly and enjoying it until approximately 1 month ago when he developed tingling and pain in his feet from the chemotherapy, which made walking more difficult. His doctor called it a neuropathy. He now cries more easily and seemingly for no good reason, such as when he sees his grandchildren playing in the yard. He wonders if he will see them grow up. He feels cognitively slowed during the past month and does not feel like socializing with friends. He easily falls asleep at night but wakes up multiple times to urinate and with hot flashes from ADT. The first couple of times he wakes up, he is able to get back to sleep easily. He is demoralized and feels like he must be depressed because he never felt like this before. He does not want to hurt himself, as that would hurt his family, but he does not want to live like this either.

Initially, John was diagnosed by his therapist as having an adjustment disorder, and he was making progress in psychotherapy. However, as his condition worsened with increased symptom burden that impaired his functioning, his mood also worsened. He did not meet full criteria for a major depression, and many of his symptoms that appeared to be related to depression could have been side effects of ADT, which eliminated his testosterone, or from chemotherapy. His likely diagnosis is now a depressive disorder due to his medical condition.

Recall from the section on medical look-a-likes that all of the physiological complaints mentioned in John's case are included in the criteria for diagnosing a major depression in a medically healthy individual without cancer. Non-prescribing clinicians need to communicate their observations and concerns to the oncology team for evaluation and possible treatment by the primary team. It is not unusual after treating a single symptom that there is still a larger depressive syndrome with multiple symptoms that needs to be addressed with an antidepressant. However, it is also important to realize that some solitary symptoms may be sufficiently upsetting and debilitating and may indeed lead to a major depressive episode if not addressed adequately.

In addition, recall the algorithm we provided to help distinguish isolated physical symptoms, such as fatigue, decreased activity, or even tearfulness, that may be direct side effects of a medication or of the cancer from a depressive episode, in which there is no sense of future orientation, hopefulness, or desire for things to get better. Now is a good time to ask those questions.

CASE: JOANNE

More Key Factors Regarding Joanne's Symptoms: Diagnosis and Etiology
Joanne's symptoms included 2 weeks of feeling down most of the day, most days. She had psychomotor slowing, poor appetite, and lost interest in activities she used to enjoy. She was tearful and had passive thoughts of dying, without acute suicidal intent or plan to hurt herself. Each of these symptoms could have been addressed individually if not viewed with a focus on depression.

But like the three blindfolded people who describe what they feel on three different parts of an elephant and cannot correctly identify the bigger picture of an elephant, we could miss the larger picture of Joanne's depressive syndrome. We should assess for cognitive slowing that may be related to past chemotherapy, fatigue, or depression and consider neurocognitive testing. Recall that Joanne stopped reading the newspaper. Was that because of her fatigue, her cognitive difficulties, or her depression? Theoretically, if her cognitive slowing or fatigue were isolated symptoms, we could treat with an activating antidepressant or a psychostimulant. But Joanne felt that life like this was not worth living: "This is not what I signed up for." Is this an isolated statement of frustration and demoralization or part of a depressive syndrome? Although people with cancer think about death, as death can be a likely outcome of cancer, most do not ruminate about it or wish it to happen, either by their own hand or by chance. The time course and severity of Joanne's constellation of symptoms (more than 2 weeks), as well as the unsuccessful resolution of symptoms with psychotherapy, would lead us to consider using an antidepressant to improve Joanne's depression. Also recall that Joanne was taking tamoxifen for her breast cancer. So, our working diagnoses, or differential diagnosis, for Joanne at this point includes a major depression and a depressive disorder due to her medical condition and possibly due to her tamoxifen therapy. Although we may not be able to determine whether Joanne's depression is due to tamoxifen treatment, a non-prescriber can discuss her syndrome with her oncology team so they can consider whether the depression should be treated simultaneously while Joanne receives tamoxifen treatment or if the tamoxifen treatment should be changed.

It is important for non-prescribing clinicians to understand how depressive symptomatology presents differently in different populations. For instance, in older people with or without cancer, depression does not always follow traditional criteria. Somatic symptoms, malaise, and gastric complaints may be common. We must all be attentive advocates for quality of life concerns because our patients sometimes take on a "grin and bear it" attitude, thinking this is what is needed in the battle against cancer. Ongoing communication with the primary oncology team can often help clarify and arrive at better outcomes more quickly.

A patient who is started on an antidepressant but who is not sleeping, like Joanne, or who is feeling anxious might be given an additional medication to address those entities for a short period of time, unless the antidepressant is known to address those symptoms. Remember that an antidepressant can take 2–6 weeks to take effect at any attempted dose. It would be a bonus for the patient to have some of their symptoms resolved while they wait for the underlying disorder to improve. So, on a short-term basis, an anxiolytic suggested for anxiety or a hypnotic, sedating medication for sleep will ease a patient's symptom burden.

THE MEDESCORT GUIDE FOR ANTIDEPRESSANTS

Metabolism of Antidepressants

As noted previously, as a non-prescriber, you do not need to know the details of drug metabolism. But the sky view bottom line is that most antidepressants are processed primarily through the liver before excretion. The medications may go through physiological processes that ultimately make them accessible to the brain to treat depression. These transformative systems may include or be mediated by proteins or enzymes in the liver (cytochrome P450 system) that may be influenced by genetic differences, liver disease, the path needed to arrive at the active metabolite of the medication, or other medications in a person's system that may compete for metabolism or accelerate the metabolism of the antidepressant. That means the antidepressant

- May get metabolized too readily, causing less than the hoped-for antidepressant effect (think of a shredder in overdrive)
  - Example
    - The antiepileptic carbamazepine will cause some antidepressants to metabolize too readily and not maintain therapeutic levels.
- May get metabolized too slowly, sluggishly, thereby accumulating in the body, causing a buildup of metabolites and possible untoward side effects
  - Example
    - Interactions with the hormonal agent abiraterone, which is used to treat prostate cancer.
- May cause the medication interacted upon to be metabolized too readily, rendering it less effective
  - Examples
    - Some antidepressants will prevent breakdown of tamoxifen to its active metabolite endoxifen, the active metabolite that has the cancer-fighting action.
    - Contraceptives for birth control or ketoconazole (an antifungal medication) used to treat prostate cancer,

which use a 3A4 mechanism of metabolism in the liver, will be less effective if combined with the wakefulness agent modafinil.

- May cause medications that have similar profiles to accumulate to toxic levels
  - Examples
    - Linezolid is an antibiotic that may be used to treat various bacterial infections, such as skin infections, as well as some infections that are resistant to other antibiotics. It is a MAOI that can increase serotonin levels and potentially lead to a toxic syndrome when combined with other medications that increase serotonin levels.
    - The hormonal agent abiraterone can interact via 2D6 liver metabolism to increase the levels of many antidepressants, potentially leading to higher than needed levels and side effects. Antidepressants commonly used in cancer settings that are potentially impacted include amitriptyline, fluoxetine, mirtazapine, nortriptyline, paroxetine, venlafaxine, and vortioxetine.
- May interact with other medications that flow through the blood strongly attached to proteins to be more available for activity
  - Examples
    - Anticoagulants such as coumadin (Warfarin) may have an increased blood-thinning effect, leading to an increased likelihood of anticoagulation, bruising, and bleeding. A prescriber of coumadin who is aware of the presence of an interacting antidepressant can readjust the daily dose of coumadin and thus the blood level of coumadin.

- Antidepressants on their own can have an impact on platelet function, potentially causing bruising and bleeding. Thus, when given with coumadin, antidepressants can increase the likelihood of anticoagulant effects.

It is likely that you will continue to see the patient for support and be able to observe for effectiveness and potential side effects once an antidepressant is started or stopped by a prescriber. It can be useful for you to help monitor the patient once an antidepressant has been started or stopped.

When to Check with the Prescriber After an Antidepressant Is Started

The following are issues that patients may raise that should be referred to prescribers:

- Does the patient have increased appetite or weight in the past few weeks or months?
    - If so, the patient can be prodded to ask the prescriber about increased glucose and/or increased weight (metabolic syndrome).
- Patients who have histories of kidney, liver, or cardiac illness abnormalities can ask their prescribers about changes in urination, limb swelling, loss of appetite, nausea, muscle aches, or chest discomfort or palpitations.
- Patients may have changes in sexual functioning since starting the antidepressant.
    - Men and women can experience decreased or delayed arousal and decreased orgasm intensity.

- Men can experience delayed orgasm/ejaculation.
- Patients can be encouraged to ask the prescriber if this may be related to the depression, the antidepressant, or some other medication, rather than just stopping the medication.
- If patients have thoughts of not wanting to be alive or to end life since starting an antidepressant, it is important to discuss this immediately with all of their providers.
  - Some of these symptoms may be related to one of their medications or a combination of their medications.
  - The non-prescriber may be the least challenging person for the patient to discuss these thoughts with and may therefore be the first responder.

In addition to recommending that the patient discuss these concerns with the prescriber, it may be helpful for you to discuss them with the treating team members directly so they can be ready to act quickly if an adverse reaction occurs. Thus, you can raise awareness about continuation or modification of antidepressant treatment as well as how those issues can best be addressed with the patient and/or family.

Potential Potholes of Antidepressant Treatment

Although antidepressants have many positive effects, there have also been reports that they may have negative consequences. Those concerns impact depressed people with or without cancer. Perhaps the most well-known alarm is that seen in television commercials for antidepressants, in which the advertisements conclude with a warning that the medications can cause the depressed person to have suicidal ideation, often referred to as a "Black Box Warning" which is placed on a prescription medication label by the Food and Drug Administration to call attention to potential serious or life-threatening side effects. This complication of suicidal ideation may be an issue in pediatric and young adult patients for whom the antidepressants were not designed. When Dr. Roth first saw those commercials, he got worried. As someone who has prescribed many antidepressants to hundreds of adults during the course of a greater than 25-year career, he had not seen such a direct path between medication and suicidal ideation as described in those commercials. On the one hand, recall that it can take weeks for an antidepressant to begin to treat depressive symptoms. That means that before the medication makes things better, the disease (depression) can get worse, and suicidal ideation, if not present earlier, may appear naturally in the course of a depressive episode. On the other hand, recall another fact about antidepressants mentioned previously: Anxiety and restlessness can be side effects of some antidepressants. Severe restlessness, also known as akathisia, might be experienced as follows: "I can't sit still. I feel like my skin is crawling" or "I feel like I am jumping out of my skin, and I cannot stand this. I want to jump out of a window." That can sound like suicidal ideation to anyone. And it is related to the antidepressant. If the potential of suicidal ideation is described in this way to patients before they start taking the medication, it may not sound as frightening because it is then an entity that is understood and can be readily managed. A non-prescriber who hears this can tell the patient,

> Let's try to contact your prescriber before you take the next dose of the antidepressant and find out what to do next—it may make sense to go to the Emergency Room to make sure you are safe. Sometimes a prescriber can recommend a medication for a few days to take away that uncomfortable feeling and help you feel better. At that point your prescriber can figure out whether you

need a different medication to treat the depression; you'll let us know if that feeling is not getting better or if it gets worse.

Unfortunately, no prescriber can predict which patient will experience any specific side effect, just as they cannot know which patients will experience the good antidepressant benefits. Prescribing clinicians cannot know who will have to try a second or different medication after an unsuccessful first trial of an antidepressant. It is no different with the prescription of any medication, whether for depression, cancer, gastric upset, Parkinson's disease, hypertension, or ulcerative colitis.

The most concerning claims against antidepressants were made in the early 1990s. There were suggestions that antidepressants were implicated in the incidence or progression of cancer. The claims have not been sufficiently confirmed in human populations. However, they have dissuaded some patients from taking these medications that might otherwise save their lives, as many might not be able to tolerate treatment for their cancer if a severe depression took hold, upturned their lives, and was not treated adequately. The original studies were done in rodents that were injected with larger amounts of tumor cells, and higher doses of antidepressants than would be used in humans. Data obtained from human participants have not supported the findings in rodents. No person should have to suffer the dual traumatic helplessness of cancer and depression.

COMMON SIDE EFFECTS OF ANTIDEPRESSANTS

It is important to inform patients about side effects before they occur. The more common side effects of antidepressants include

---

Box 1.7 THE NOT-SO-GOOD SIDE EFFECTS OF NEWER
ANTIDEPRESSANTS (SSRIS, SNRIS, AND DOPAMINE
REUPTAKE INHIBITORS)

- Gastric distress
- Headaches
- Sedation or insomnia
- Weight gain or loss with metabolic syndrome
- Sexual dysfunction
- Dry mouth still a possibility

---

gastric upset, daytime sluggishness, anxiety or restlessness, and in-somnia (Box 1.7). These side effects are not dangerous and can often be avoided by the prescriber starting at lower doses than usual and titrating (increasing) the medication slowly to the therapeutic dose.

You can confirm the likelihood that your patient's complaints are related to the medication, another medication, or perhaps some-thing entirely different. Hearing from you that it is important to check with the prescriber helps assure the patient that they will not be a nuisance or viewed as a "complainer," as many patients fear.

Gastric Upset

Most of the antidepressants developed in the past 30 years can cause gastric upset—that is, bloating, nausea, constipation, or diarrhea—more commonly at the start of treatment. If a patient gets any of these, they can be reassured that the side effect is likely to improve in approximately 1 or 2 weeks. However, the intensity or frequency of the symptom could be a deal breaker. After a few days, we titrate the dose up slowly to a target goal, hoping that the patient will become tolerant to the side effects again and can wait for the wanted antidepressant effects to begin. The only contemporary antidepressant not likely to cause gastric upset is mirtazapine. Most people find that they have fewer gastric side effects if they take the medication after a meal, not on an empty stomach.

Sluggishness or Fatigue

Patients who are already bothered or depressed by fatigue because of cancer or cancer treatment do not need another medication to worsen that fatigue; some antidepressants can cause sleepiness even at lower doses. In fact, a patient complaining of fatigue might seem confused if a prescriber recommends a psychostimulant medication to improve energy; after all, that is what their child or grandchild took for attention-deficit/hyperactivity disorder and it appeared to calm them down. Similarly, a patient may be baffled if the antidepressant bupropion is suggested for fatigue; it can have an invigorating, stimulant side effect to alleviate fatigue. It works on the dopamine neurotransmitter system and is safe if the patient does not have a history of seizures or bulimia (Table 1.2).

Table 1.2 Bupropion: Multiple Birds with One Antidepressant

Advantages	Disadvantages
Improves mood	May cause anxiety, agitation,
Smoking cessation	and insomnia
Counters fatigue with activating effects	May aggravate psychotic
Does not cause any sexual side effects	symptoms
like other antidepressants might	May lower seizure threshold

A major difficulty in choosing any medication is that there is no crystal ball to know who might develop which side effects, if any, at what intensity, or the degree of interference the side effects might play in their daily routines. Our strategy of starting these antidepressants at lower than usual dosages often allows for awareness of and adjustment to the more common symptoms, and it permits the body to adapt and develop tolerance for whichever side effects may arise.

Drug Interactions

Additional serious side effects to be aware of that prescribers try to avoid include mixing two medications that have serotonergic side effects that may result in a serotonin syndrome caused by excessive serotonergic activity. Complications of serotonin syndrome include agitation, high blood pressure, confusion, increased reflexes, tremor, muscle twitching, sweating, diarrhea, coma, and death. For instance, patients who are on a serotonergic medication can be at risk if another serotonergic medication, or an MAOI that increases serotonin levels is added. Therefore, if meperidine or toradol (pain medications) or procarbazine (a chemotherapy agent) are added to the regimen of a patient already on an SSRI for any indication, levels of serotonin can build up and lead to a dangerous outcome. Depending on the SSRI, there may need to be a 2-week or longer washout period prior to starting procarbazine, depending on the half-life of the SSRI (how long it takes to metabolize and ultimately leave the body). Other medications that can cause these interactions in cancer patients include, but are not limited to, linezolid, methadone, dextromethorphan, and sumatriptan.

If the patient is taking an antipsychotic along with a serotonergic antidepressant, prescribers and non-prescribing clinicians should be aware of two major, although rare, complications that can be life-threatening and that must be distinguished from each other: serotonin syndrome, caused by an excess of serotonin, and neuroleptic malignant syndrome, caused by an antipsychotic-related hypodopaminergic state (complications include rigidity, hyperthermia, confusion, unstable blood pressure, variable heart rate, and other autonomic anomalies). The prescriber will stop the potentially problematic medications and consider intensive medical monitoring of the patient and appropriate intervention.

One must also always consider the patient's psychiatric history. Any patient who has had a manic episode or hypomania in the past may be at risk of developing mania from antidepressant treatment. Primary prescribers may not readily receive this information. If you have elicited this information in your psychological history when you started treatment with the patient, it is useful to pass it on to the prescriber.

THE OLDER ANTIDEPRESSANTS

Tricyclic Antidepressants: Amitriptyline, Imipramine, Nortriptyline, and Desipramine

Tricyclic antidepressants were introduced in the 1950s and were the mainstay of the pharmacologic treatment of depression until the 1990s when the SSRIs became available (Table 1.3). Unfortunately, the uncomfortable or potentially dangerous side effects of TCAs include dry mouth, blurry vision, constipation, difficulty urinating, sedation that often leads to falls, cardiac conduction problems, abnormal heart rhythms, and blood pressure changes, which make them particularly problematic for medically or physically susceptible adults with cancer, especially the elderly. Today, these medications

Table 1.3 The Basics About Medications to Treat Depression

Drug Class, Generic Name (Brand Name)	Starting Dose (Start Low, Go Slowly)	Non-Psycho-Oncologist Sky View: Pearls and Potholes
Antidepressants		Be aware of potential drug interactions with all other medications.
SSRIs		
Citalopram (Celexa)	10 mg daily	Varying degrees of gastric distress, nausea, headache, insomnia, sweating, increased anxiety, and sexual dysfunction. In general, sertraline, citalopram, and escitalopram produce the least drug–drug interactions. In addition to treating depression, these medications are used for anxiety and panic syndromes as well as off-label hot flashes.
Escitalopram (Lexapro)	5–10 mg daily	
Fluoxetine (Prozac)	10 mg daily	
Paroxetine (Paxil)	10 mg daily	
Sertraline (Zoloft)	12.5–25 mg daily	
Vortioxetine (Trintillex)	5–10 mg daily	
SNRIs		
Venlafaxine (Effexor)	25–37.5 mg daily	These medications also treat anxiety and panic syndromes, in addition to off-label hot flashes. Slow or extended-release venlafaxine decreases likelihood of raising blood pressure.
Desvenlafaxine (Pristiq)	50 mg daily	
Duloxetine (Cymbalta)	30–60 mg daily	

Drug	Dosage	Comments
Milnacipran (Ixel, Savella, Dalcipran, Toledomin)	12.5 titrated to 50 mg daily over 1 week	Duloxetine may help with neuropathic pain syndromes and fibromyalgia. Milnacipran is more often used for fibromyalgia and other pain syndromes. Side effects include varying degrees of activation, gastric distress, nausea, anxiety, sedation, and sweating.
Other antidepressants		
Mirtazapine (Remeron)	7.5–15 mg daily at bedtime	No gastric side effects. Can improve sleep and appetite but may cause unwanted daytime sedation or weight gain. Dissolvable tablet form available—no swallowing needed.
Bupropion (Wellbutrin)	100 mg SR daily	Activating: helps fatigue but can cause anxiety, restlessness, or insomnia. May cause seizures if predisposed, or when combined with alcohol or with sudden weight loss, as with bulimia. Helps with smoking cessation. No sexual side effects

SNRIs, serotonin norepinephrine reuptake inhibitors; SR, slow release; SSRIs, selective serotonin reuptake inhibitors.

are used to treat chronic neuropathic pain syndromes and occasionally insomnia, but they are seldom used as first-line medications to treat depression. Although SSRIs and SNRIs are used more commonly, TCAs can be helpful in some treatment-resistant patients.

Today, you will likely see few or no patients on the oldest of the antidepressants—TCAs—but it is still important to be knowledgeable about them (Table 1.4). They are more commonly prescribed by neurologists for the treatment of headaches or neuropathic pain syndromes, by gastroenterologists for irritable bowel syndrome, or by the psycho-oncology prescriber in low doses to help with sleep (e.g., doxepin). TCAs are still used to manage difficult-to-treat depressive syndromes that do not respond to the newer first-line antidepressants. Being knowledgeable about these less commonly used antidepressants, you and your patients may more fully appreciate the newer medications.

Table 1.4 Tricyclic Antidepressants

TCA	Starting Dose (Start Low, Go Slowly)	Non-Psycho-Oncologist Sky View: Pearls and Potholes
Amitriptyline (Elavil)	10–25 mg hs; increasing by 10–25 mg every few days	Have baseline ECG and monitor regularly. Monitor BP, HR, and orthostatic BPs. Monitor constipation, dry mouth, and urinary retention. Blood levels can be drawn after initiating TCA treatment. These levels can help assess toxicity.

Table 1.4 Continued

TCA	Starting Dose (Start Low, Go Slowly)	Non-Psycho-Oncologist Sky View: Pearls and Potholes
Imipramine (Tofranil)	10–25 mg hs; increasing by 10–25 mg every 1–2 weeks	Have baseline ECG and monitor regularly. Monitor BP, HR, and orthostatic BPs. Monitor constipation, dry mouth, and urinary retention. Blood levels can be useful to assess toxicity.
Nortriptyline (Pamelor)	10–25 mg hs; increase as tolerated to 30–50 mg hs	Blood levels for nortriptyline are unique in that they not only help assess toxicity but also can provide a therapeutic window, below and above which the medication will not treat depression. Less ACh than amitriptyline and imipramine.
Desipramine (Norpramin)	25–50 mg daily; may be titrated as needed (up to 150 mg daily for older patients)	Have baseline ECG and monitor regularly. No ACh side effects. May be less sedating than other TCAs.

ACh, anticholinergic; BP, blood pressure; ECG, electrocardiogram; HR, heart rate; TCAs, tricyclic antidepressants.

Monoamine Oxidase Inhibitors

SOME ANTIDEPRESSANTS JUST DON'T CUT IT IN CANCER

The antidepressants from this class of medications are not used frequently anymore, especially in people with cancer. The original MAOI medications phenelzine (Nardil), tranylcypromine (Parnate), and isocarboxazid (Marplan) were excellent medications in terms of antidepressant benefits, especially in patients with depressions resistant to other treatment. They were also helpful to those who had atypical depressions—that is, those who had increased sleep, increased appetite and weight, reversed diurnal variation of mood (e.g., they felt better in the morning), transient mood improvements with positive events, more intense reactivity to rejection, had a weighted down or leaden feeling, and/or experienced social withdrawal. The problem with these medications was their severe side effect profiles that included many of the same problems that the TCAs had (i.e., orthostasis or positional changes in blood pressure, cardiac conduction problems, and sedation) but also significant dietary restrictions for fear of a dangerous interaction with foods that contained tyramine. This interaction could cause a hypertensive crisis that could cause headache; palpitations; and possible complications of stroke, cardiac arrhythmias, cardiac failure, or death. Notorious foods that could bring on these reactions included aged cheeses, cured meats, pickled or fermented foods, fava beans, and alcoholic beverages such as beer or Chianti. People with cancer already have significant restrictions on quality of life. They might find these additional dietary restrictions even more challenging and anxiety-provoking. MAOI antidepressants could also interact with other medications such as the opioid Demerol, the antibiotic linezolid, the chemotherapy agent procarbazine, as well as the SSRI and SNRI antidepressants, potentially causing dangerous hypertensive or serotonergic crises. Thus, their use has been shunned for medically healthy depressed people since newer and safer antidepressants have become available, and particularly in depressed cancer patients. For example, the MAOI medication selegiline (Emsam), used in the treatment of Parkinson's disease, is safer and has no dietary restrictions.

The Older Antidepressants Can Cause Anticholinergic Side Effects

There is an old ditty to help remember anticholinergic side effects caused by many classes of medications: Blind as a bat, mad as a hatter, red as a beet, hot as a hare, dry as a bone, bowel and bladder tone, and the heart runs alone.

If your patient complains of blurred vision, confusion, flushing, sweating, fast heart rate, dry mouth, difficulty urinating, or constipation, think "anticholinergic side effects" and wonder about the timeline from prescription to side effect emergence (Figure 1.7). Then suggest that the patient call their prescriber to check.

The patient may be on more than one medication that could cause anticholinergic side effects, which could increase the likelihood of experiencing them. For instance, an antihistamine such as diphenhydramine (Benadryl) or an antiemetic such as prochlorperazine (Compazine) or metoclopramide (Reglan) can have similar side effects that may be unnoticed when only one medication is taken, but compounded when there are two or more on board. Therefore, if your patient is getting a TCA such as amitriptyline for sleep or for a neuropathic pain syndrome and starts to complain of constipation, it could be caused by the amitriptyline alone or the addition of another medication with similar side effects.

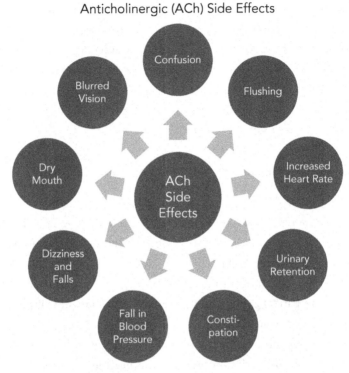

Figure 1.7. Anticholinergic (Ach) side effects.

Tricyclic Antidepressants Can Cause Orthostatic Hypotension

The older antidepressants also cause dangerous side effects, including dropping blood pressure, especially when people change positions, such as from lying down to sitting or from sitting to standing up. This is called orthostatic hypotension, which can cause dizziness and falls, possibly leading to fractures such as broken hips or concussions in older patients.

The non-prescribing clinician can suggest "fall-prevention and safety tips" prophylactically to the patients, but also suggest

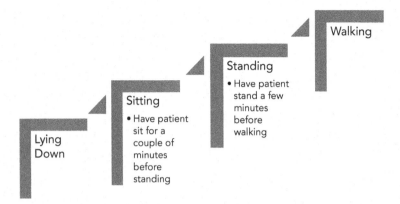

Figure 1.8. Safety tips for medications that can cause orthostatic hypotension (Tricyclics, MAOIs).

the patient contact the prescriber should these symptoms occur (Figure 1.8):

- When getting out of bed, don't stand right away.
  - Sit up for a minute or two before standing.
  - When going from sitting to standing position, don't start walking immediately—just stand for a few minutes to increase the likelihood of steadiness.
  - Encourage sufficient hydration.

Tricyclic Antidepressants Can Cause Sedation

These older antidepressants are often sedating. They help patients get to sleep and stay asleep at night but may leave people feeling groggy and cloudy during the day. This side effect also contributes to falls, especially in older people.

Tricyclic Antidepressants Can Cause Cardiac Conduction Abnormalities

This side effect was one of the greatest concerns for prescribers. Patients with significant cardiac histories were often not allowed to take a TCA for fear of causing an arrhythmia or severe slowing of the heart conduction. An electrocardiogram (ECG) would be taken before treatment was started and would be monitored regularly for rate and rhythm abnormalities.

The cardiac side effects of TCAs could be dangerous in any patient. Patients would start to feel better on these medications, recognize how badly they had been feeling emotionally or the challenging circumstances that might have made them feel depressed in the first place, and overdose on the medications in serious or successful suicide attempts, dying of a lethal cardiac arrhythmia. Therefore, when we prescribed these medications for depression or neuropathic pain syndromes in the past, we would often not give even a month's worth of the medication to some patients, concerned about a suicide attempt with the medication we prescribed to ease someone's suffering. We would request that the patient return for the next prescription in 1 or 2 weeks for safety's sake.

As shown in Boxes 1.8–1.10, the older antidepressants have a very different, and more dangerous, set of potential complications—anticholinergic, blood pressure, orthostatic

---

Box 1.8 SECONDARY USES FOR OLDER ANTIDEPRESSANTS
(TRICYCLICS, MAOIS)

The older antidepressants may still be prescribed to treat neuropathic pain syndromes, headaches, insomnia, irritable bowel syndrome, or resistant major depression (that does not respond to a newer antidepressant).

Box 1.9 COMMON SIDE EFFECTS OF OLDER ANTIDEPRESSANTS (TRICYCLICS, MAOIS)

- Anticholinergic
  - Blurry vision, confusion, flushing, sweating, dry mouth, difficulty urinating or constipation, tachycardia (an increase in heart rate that can cause palpitations)
- Orthostatic hypotension
  - Significant changes in blood pressure (dropping) or heart rate (increasing) with changes in position from lying or sitting to sitting or standing
- Sedation
- Cardiac conduction problems (ECG):
  - Usually a slowing of electric transmission that regulates heart rate and rhythm

---

hypotension, tachycardia, cardiac conduction slowing that can lead to arrhythmia, and sedation. For the most part, the newer antidepressants—the SSRIs, DRIs, and SNRIs—may have what we would call discomfort complications, such as gastric upset,

---

Box 1.10 DOWNSTREAM EFFECTS OF THE OLD WAY WITH TCAS

- Falls
- Confusion
- Cardiac abnormalities
- Overdose and suicide potential

---

anxiety, weight gain, insomnia or restlessness, or sexual problem. Often, lowering the dose of the medication or starting a different medication can resolve these problems. Sometimes adding a second medication for a brief period can help resolve anxiety, insomnia, or fatigue. The second medication can then be withdrawn after the antidepressant has had time to achieve its mood-elevating effects.

Sexual Side Effects

One of the most aversive, yet common, side effects of the SSRIs or SNRIs is sexual dysfunction, which generally includes reduction in sexual interest and extended orgasm latency. Although this is a frequent side effect that leads to medication discontinuation in medically healthy people, it does not appear to be as problematic in those with cancer who may have lower libido from some of the other medications they receive for their treatment. It is important for the non-prescriber to discuss this symptom if it occurs to guide the patient through challenges to intimacy in close relationships and, if related to the antidepressant, to discuss a possible change with the prescriber.

SAFETY CONSIDERATIONS

Remember Potential Contraindications and Drug Interactions

There may be several prescribers involved with one patient's care, and sometimes, too many cooks can inadvertently cause trouble. Home medication lists are only as good as the patient or caregiver who is monitoring or overseeing them. Communication between prescribers is vital, although sometimes the only communication link between all prescribers is the patient, especially if prescribers are at different institutions without access to the same medical chart. The non-prescriber can be the glue that keeps the treatment puzzle pieces together.

Pertinent history can help a prescriber with medication choice. For instance, bupropion is not a good antidepressant to give someone who has a susceptibility to seizures. It is therefore also not a good medication to give someone who is already on another medication that can also make someone prone to seizures. So, if one prescriber is suggesting bupropion for depression or smoking cessation, and another prescriber has already recommended enzalutamide for prostate cancer, you as the non-prescriber can at least ask the reasonable question of both prescribers: "Is the potential risk of an interaction that can cause seizures worth the benefit?" It may be, but all should go into this with awareness and agreement.

The same is true for a woman with breast cancer who is depressed and is taking tamoxifen (Box 1.11). An outside prescriber suggests an antidepressant. Although the literature is still controversial regarding the degree to which the interactions between some antidepressants and tamoxifen interfere with the breakdown of tamoxifen to its active cancer-fighting metabolite endoxifen, with a potential impact on cancer control, there are safer choices. If you hear recommendations for venlafaxine, desvenlafaxine, citalopram, escitalopram, or mirtazapine, you can feel more comfortable. If you hear suggestions for bupropion, fluoxetine, or paroxetine, you can voice your concern about possible P450 2D6 interactions.

Box 1.11 CONCERN ABOUT ANTIDEPRESSANTS IN WOMEN
ON TAMOXIFEN

- Liver enzyme activity may adversely affect tamoxifen metabolism.
  - Inhibited breakdown to active endoxifen metabolite.
  - Avoid antidepressants that are more likely culprits in this process:
    - Fluoxetine (Prozac), paroxetine (Paxil), bupropion (Wellbutrin), and fluvoxamine (Luvox)
  - Consider antidepressants that are less likely to inhibit tamoxifen's benefits:
    - Venlafaxine (Effexor), desvenlafaxine (Pristiq) mirtazapine (Remeron), citalopram (Celexa), and escitalopram (Lexapro)
- Consideration could be given to potential genetic susceptibility for aberrant liver metabolism or to finding an alternative hormonal treatment for breast cancer.

UNDERSTANDING THE STRATEGIES OF THE PSYCHO-ONCOLOGY MEDICATION PRESCRIBER

How a Prescriber Thinks About Prescribing an Antidepressant Medication

We have noted that all antidepressants are supposedly equally efficacious for treating depression. But they do not work for all patients all the time. And sometimes the unknown biochemistry of one person's depression will require linking to a specific type of antidepressant or dose of a particular medication. Some patients cannot tolerate the side effects of a medication, whereas some side effects work in the patient's favor. So, psycho-oncology prescribers develop strategies to choose medications they believe might be right for the situation, even though there is no way to know for sure what the right medication for a patient would be. That is why it is good for prescribers to be comfortable with antidepressants from various groups.

Boxes 1.12 and 1.13 indicate how psycho-oncology prescribers might assess the patient's current condition and what side effects might be helpful, or improve, the patient's current physical and emotional well-being.

If your patient is depressed about a recent lung cancer diagnosis and feels helpless to stop her lifelong tobacco habit, you can mention the use of bupropion for smoking cessation. It

---

Box 1.12 QUESTIONS TO CONSIDER FOR CHOOSING THE
"RIGHT" ANTIDEPRESSANT

Are there additional actions or side effects beyond the stated benefit of treating depression?

Can an antidepressant maximize benefits or minimize discomfort on the patient's review of symptoms?

Are there P450 interactions to be aware of?

Is there a personal or family history of antidepressant success?

Is there a history of manic or hypomanic episodes?

Box 1.13 QUESTIONS ABOUT ANTIDEPRESSANT TWOFERS—
WITH SOLUTIONS

Is the patient having trouble falling asleep?

If yes, does the patient get to sleep fine but wakes up
often in the middle of the night?

If they do, is it because they have other physical
symptoms such as pain, urinary frequency,
cough, or gastric upset? These symptoms need
to be addressed medically if possible. Sedating
someone enough to sleep through a physical
issue can be helpful but could also lead to a wet
bed or one full of feces in the morning.

Can consider sedating antidepressants such as
mirtazapine or trazodone or a benzo or an
atypical antipsychotic such as olanzapine or
quetiapine.

Does the patient get back to sleep within 20–30 minutes of
awakening?

If yes, no medication needed. May try relaxation or visualization techniques and reviewing sleep hygiene.

Is the patient eating well?

Is there no or low appetite or a decrease or change
in taste?

Consider an appetite stimulant such as megestrol,
dronabinol, or a steroid; an antidepressant such
as mirtazapine; or an atypical antipsychotic such

as olanzapine, all of which may increase appetite
mirtazapine or an antidepressant such as olanzapine.
Does the patient have a neuropathic pain syndrome?
Consider duloxetine, milnacipran, or a TCA.
Does the patient have daytime fatigue or trouble
staying awake?
Consider a stimulating antidepressant such as bupropion or a psychostimulant.
Is the patient having difficulty concentrating?
Consider neurocognitive testing or brain imaging to en-
sure there is no medical cause from cancer or cancer
treatment (i.e., chemotherapy, radiation therapy, or
opioids).
Consider a psychostimulant or bupropion (which is
sometimes given to children with attention-deficit/
hyperactivity disorder to help with concentration).
Avoid some antidepressants with anticholinergic side
effects (i.e., TCAs).
Does the patient have hot flashes that awaken them frequently at night?
Consider SSRI, SNRI, or adding gabapentin.
Is the patient feeling anxious?
Consider mirtazapine or a short-term benzodiazepine
or atypical antipsychotic such as olanzapine or
quetiapine.

works on dopaminergic transmitters, which are active players in the reward center in the brain. A common side effect is anxiety, which is not helpful when someone is trying to eliminate an emotional crutch they have been using for years. Bupropion can aide smoking cessation even if the patient does not have depression. But if started at a lower than usual dose and titrated to the therapeutic dose, it may be a good adjuvant to the treatment you are doing with the patient. In addition, you could recommend that the patient see a smoking cessation counselor for assistance or other options, such as nicotine replacement treatment.

OUR CASELOAD—ANTIDEPRESSANT CHOICES

CASE: JOANNE

Choosing an Antidepressant

Joanne has many symptoms of depression, including a few weeks of depressed mood and tearfulness. We could try to treat her symptoms individually if we did not see the bigger picture of a major depression. We could treat anxiety and worry (fear of recurrence) with an antianxiety medication. Ongoing thoughts about how life is not worth living, even without an active suicidal plan or intent to hurt oneself, as in Joanne's case, are likely part of a depressive syndrome rather than an isolated symptom.

Joanne's breast cancer regimen consists of tamoxifen. That means the antidepressant chosen by the prescriber should have the least interactions with tamoxifen, as the last thing the psychotropic prescriber wants to do is inadvertently decrease the effectiveness of the cancer treatment. If there were no other options, the prescriber might discuss the possibility of changing the tamoxifen treatment to another aromatase inhibitor. However, venlafaxine, desvenlafaxine, mirtazapine, and citalopram are reasonable medication options that are much less likely to inhibit the metabolism of tamoxifen to its active metabolite, endoxifen, and would be much safer to use.

Joanne's low appetite might be boosted by a medication such as mirtazapine, which is considered relatively safe with tamoxifen. Olanzapine or a psychostimulant might also be considered relatively safe if the prescriber wanted to treat the low appetite with either of those medications; however, of these three medications, only mirtazapine would treat the full depressive spectrum. In terms of Joanne being less active and more socially isolated, we can ask what she would do if she had more energy and felt clearer cognitively. If she mentioned activities she would like to do, lowering the likelihood of a major depressive syndrome, we could treat her lethargy and apathy with a psychostimulant or an energizing antidepressant such as bupropion, although bupropion has strong liver interactions with tamoxifen. But Joanne, who does have an ongoing depressive episode, is likely to answer, "It doesn't matter, I don't really care." It would still be necessary to recommend behavioral activation, but that would be insufficient to treat the depressive syndrome. Both the prescriber and the non-prescriber would need to monitor Joanne's energy if the chosen antidepressant is mirtazapine. Although mirtazapine can help with sleep, some patients will feel more tired during the day from a possible "hangover" effect. Alternatively, the prescriber could consider a more neutral antidepressant that would not target any specific quality-of-life symptoms (fatigue, insomnia, and appetite) but would be as effective to treat the major depression and not interfere with tamoxifen metabolism. These medications could include venlafaxine, desvenlafaxine, citalopram, or escitalopram.

If Joanne were taken off tamoxifen by her oncologist, the prescribing options change. Prescribers could consider an activating antidepressant, such as bupropion, to address fatigue and low appetite, in addition to treating the depression. They need to recognize that any activating medication could make anxiety, worry, or insomnia worse. We could choose a sedating antidepressant such as mirtazapine, which could address sleeplessness, low appetite, and anxiety, in addition to eventually treating the depressive episode, but it could potentially make daytime energy worse in the short term. Or we could choose an SSRI or an SNRI that has less potential to help with energy or calm but also less potential for overshoot side effects of anxiety, insomnia, or drowsiness. The prescriber could add a psychostimulant, which tends to work immediately, to one of the non-energizing antidepressants for a few weeks to give Joanne a more immediate effect. Alternatively, a benzodiazepine such as clonazepam could help with sleep and/or anxiety until the antidepressant has a chance to be effective.

CASE: JAKE

Choosing an Antidepressant

Jake became depressed after recurrence of his lung cancer. He had a depressed mood, anhedonia, hopelessness, and social withdrawal. He did not have neurovegetative signs of changes in appetite or energy or sleep. There were no secondary benefits to gain from exploiting or avoiding any side effects. A prescriber could consider just about any antidepressant. The neutral antidepressants such as escitalopram, sertraline, and venlafaxine, do not clearly favor any specific side effect profiles, such as sedation for insomnia, or energizing for fatigue, and may therefore more easily coexist with other medications and hopefully be easily tolerated. In this case, Jake's prescriber chose escitalopram. In follow-up sessions, Jake's non-prescribing therapist was able to make sure Jake was taking the medication as prescribed and was not having any side effects. The therapist was also able to continue encouraging behavioral activation and engagement in social activities, even though the activities felt like an endless mountain climb that Jake would rather avoid. In the therapist's words, "Jake, initially, you need to fake it until you make it. When the medication kicks in, you will no longer be faking it."

CASE: JOHN

Choosing an Antidepressant

The therapist relayed to John's prescribers that John's psychiatric diagnosis had transitioned from an adjustment disorder to a depressive disorder due to medical condition, likely related to his androgen deprivation therapy and chemotherapy. His prescribers can now think about giving him gabapentin or pregabalin, which could help his neuropathy, hot flashes, and sleep, as they can also be sedating. However, neither of these medications is likely to help his depression. The prescribers might consider duloxetine, which is an SNRI, for his depression. Duloxetine can help mood, anxiety, and neuropathy. At this point, non-prescribers will still encourage behavioral activation, help John understand the benefits of the antidepressant, and reinforce taking it regularly. The non-prescribing clinicians can also deal with the tensions and concerns about John becoming more dependent on others and the potential benefits of continuing with physical therapy while still needing to care for his wife, who also has physical limitations. They can also help John consider practical options for assistance with his wife's home care needs. A therapist may also help John deal with his concerns about dying and how to live a meaningful life with purpose even with the shortcomings brought on by cancer.

PSYCHOSTIMULANTS

Psychostimulants can treat symptoms of depression and fatigue as well as foggy concentration and sedating side effects of other medications used in people with cancer (Table 1.5), and are discussed in greater detail in Chapter 5 on Medications for Fatigue. The more common

Table 1.5 Potential Benefits of Psychostimulants

Syndrome	Potential Benefits
Depression	Improved mood, interest, and motivation to do pleasurable activities; improved sense of well-being
Cognitive deficits from cancer treatment	Improved attention and focused concentration
Neuropathic pain	Adjuvant analgesia; may potentiate opioid effects
Sedation due to opioids	May improve alertness and energy
Fatigue, weakness, and decreased motivation	May improve energy and motivation to participate in behavioral activation, increasing strength/stamina
Poor appetite	May increase activity and secondarily appetite

stimulants include amphetamines and methylphenidate. These medications were abused in the 1960s and 1970s as diet pills and as "uppers" to help students stay awake longer to study more. Today, they are among the armamentarium to help children and adults who have attention-deficit/hyperactivity disorder because they help sharpen alertness and concentration. Early on, clinicians were concerned about decreasing appetite and worsening dietary intake in cancer patients who were already troubled by nausea and gastric upset. Studies have been inconsistent in showing the extent of benefits of low doses of psychostimulants to increase energy, activity, and appetite in medically ill patients, but our experience has shown that psychostimulants are worth a try depending on the individual situation and safety concerns. The rule of thumb we use to start antidepressants is true for psychostimulants as well: *Start at low dosages and titrate slowly*. If effects overshoot into side effects, people can feel anxious, irritable, and have trouble sleeping. Methylphenidate and amphetamines are relatively contraindicated in patients who have a history of seizures or cardiac arrhythmias, so a patient's cardiologist or neurologist should approve their use. A newer, gentler stimulant such as modafinil does not have such contraindications and appears to be much safer and can often be tolerated better by people with cancer.

The Dosing of Psychostimulants: Starting Low, Going Slowly . . . Again

The dosing of psychostimulants as well as the sky view pearls and potholes are highlighted in Table 1.6. Methylphenidate or the amphetamines would be started at 2.5 mg in the morning and, if necessary, can be increased by 2.5 mg in the morning and/or early afternoon every 2 or 3 days until a good effect is seen. These medications can ease the fatigue caused by cancer and cancer treatments such as radiation therapy, chemotherapy, and pain medications. If a dose of an immediate-release stimulant does not last long enough, extended-release or longer acting medications can be used. Modafinil would be started at 50–100 mg in the morning and may be increased to 50 mg in the morning and in the early afternoon if needed. Problems arise when clinicians start doses too high or do not increase the medications sufficiently because of fear of addiction.

Table 1.6 The Psychostimulants

Psychostimulants	Starting Dose (Start Low, Go Slowly)	Non-Psychiatrist Sky View Focus: Pearls and Potholes
Methylphenidate (Ritalin; Focalin) Amphetamine (Adderall)	2.5–5 mg in the morning (can be taken with early afternoon dose)	Psychostimulants can improve mood, energy, concentration, and appetite.
	2.5–5 mg in the morning (can be taken with early afternoon dose)	Possible cardiac rhythm complications or hypertension; seizures if predisposed; agitation, restlessness, anxiety, insomnia, and tics can occur.
	50–100 mg daily in the morning	Titrate the dose as needed for improved energy and minimized side effects. Vyvanse is expensive and may not be covered by insurance.
Modafinil, armodafinil (Provigil; Nuvigil)		Wakefulness agents. Usually well tolerated. Improve energy, mood, and focus. These are expensive and not covered by many prescription plans. Side effects include nausea, anxiety, insomnia, and increased heart rate.

TREATMENT ALGORITHM FOR DEPRESSIVE SYNDROMES

Looking for antidepressant response: 4- to 6-week trial of an
SSRI at any one dose

The medication will be titrated until efficacious every
4–6 weeks.

If no response at maximum dose, another SSRI or SNRI
will be tried. The first medication will be tapered off or
discontinued.

If a partial response is seen, an adjunct medication, such
as mirtazapine or bupropion, can be added to optimize
the SSRI.

Looking for additional benefits (i.e., to help sleep, energy, or
appetite)

If the patient's depression is accompanied by significant anxiety or insomnia, we may start a neutral antidepressant that does not have a sedating side effect along with a benzodiazepine or trazodone to help with anxiety or sleep. If the patient's anxious depression is accompanied by severe ruminations, we may give the antidepressant with an atypical antipsychotic, such as olanzapine or quetiapine. If the patient's depression includes significant fatigue or apathy, we may start the antidepressant with a psychostimulant.

For patients who may be nearing end of life, we may skip the antidepressant and use a faster acting psychostimulant for both mood and energy (Figure 1.9).

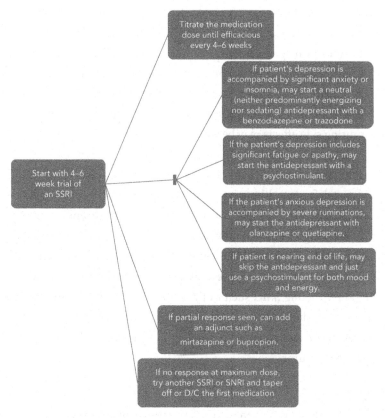

Figure 1.9. Treating depressive syndromes in people with cancer.

A FINAL WORD ABOUT ANTIDEPRESSANTS: DISCONTINUATION PEARLS AND POTHOLES

When a patient has been on an antidepressant for more than a few weeks and the antidepressant is to be discontinued, the antidepressant should be tapered over days or weeks to prevent a discontinuation syndrome or withdrawal. An antidepressant that has been effective may be discontinued after 9–12 months of successful treatment. If the depressive symptoms recur, the antidepressant can be restarted. An antidepressant that is found to be ineffective or is causing side effects may be stopped sooner.

Discontinuation syndrome can be extremely uncomfortable, especially with the shorter acting SSRIs, venlafaxine, and desvenlafaxine. Although potentially highly distressing, it should be emphasized to patients that discontinuation syndrome is not life-threatening. Patients may experience body aches, malaise, or flu-like symptoms. They may also feel dizzy or experience electric shock-like pains (Box 1.14). A prescriber might slow the taper; substitute a longer acting SSRI such as fluoxetine to ease the discomfort; or provide a short-term prescription of a benzodiazepine, such as lorazepam or clonazepam, to relieve the side effects that arise with discontinuation.

Box 1.14 THE ANNOYING SYMPTOMS OF DISCONTINUATION SYNDROME

- Malaise or flu-like symptoms
- Dizziness
- Electric shock-like pains in head or extremities

NON-PRESCRIBER QUESTIONS ABOUT ANTIDEPRESSANT TREATMENT

Q: My patient with depression was started on sertraline 25 mg daily by her primary care doctor. The antidepressant dose was increased to 50 mg after 5 days. The patient said she felt better in a week. Is that possible, if it takes 2–6 weeks for an antidepressant to "kick in"?

A: Yes. It is possible, especially if the patient is getting a secondary benefit from a side effect. For instance, the medication may be having a sedating effect that aids sleep or an energizing effect that eases fatigue or lethargy. However, because the reason for improvement is not definitively clear, the patient should stay on sertraline to potentially experience more of its benefits as time progresses.

Q: I am referring my patient to the psychiatrist for antidepressant treatment. The patient has colorectal cancer and unsettled bowel regulation. Ten years ago, she was treated with sertraline for depression prior to surgery. Is that a good medication to start with again?

A: On the one hand, the prescriber might want to use a medication that has been tried and was successful 10 years ago. On the other hand, sertraline as well as the other SSRIs and SNRIs can have bowel side effects. So, prescribers might start with low doses and see if tolerated. If not tolerated, they might consider mirtazapine as an alternative.

Q: I have been doing occupational therapy with my patient, a 53-year-old man with metastatic lung cancer. He has smoked heavily for 35 years and would like to stop smoking. He has made several quit dates but has not succeeded. His mood is down, he is fatigued, but it is not clear that he is depressed. He does not like taking medications. Does it make sense to refer him to a psychotropic prescriber?

A: Yes, it does. He may be a good candidate for bupropion. It can help many people stop smoking, and if his mood is related to a major depressive episode, it will help with that as well. If his fatigue is just fatigue, bupropion can elevate energy in the short term.

Q: I am a nurse for a 48-year-old woman treated for breast cancer with surgery and chemotherapy. She complains of feeling washed out during the day, although she sleeps well at night. She finds it difficult to multitask at her job as a bookkeeper. The change in her productivity has had a negative effect on her self-esteem. She is sexually active but does not seem to enjoy sex as much anymore. The patient has struggled with body image changes as well as trying to find enjoyable activities that might match her low energy, but it seems like she has hit a wall. What would a prescriber be able to offer?

A: The patient may benefit from a psychostimulant to help with cognition and energy. It is possible that bupropion could help with that as well. In fact, bupropion is one of the only antidepressants that will not interfere with sexual functioning. Of course, in order to utilize bupropion, the patient should not have a history of seizures or bulimia. Similarly, there should be no history of an arrhythmia in a patient to whom the prescriber is considering giving a psychostimulant, such as methylphenidate or an amphetamine. It might be safer for her to take modafinil or armodafinil if she has a history of seizures. However, bupropion would be a problematic choice if the patient is on tamoxifen for her breast cancer.

Q: My patient is a 79-year-old man with recurrent metastatic kidney cancer who has been demoralized for approximately 6 months. He was treated for depression approximately 40 years ago with amitriptyline, which worked well. He complains of weakness, fatigue, and trouble sleeping. He says, "I can't even do my work projects around the house. I feel so incompetent." He has atrial fibrillation and an enlarged prostate with difficulty urinating, so I am not sure if he can tolerate an antidepressant. Should I just keep trying with psychotherapy to try to help him?

A: Keep the psychotherapy going. It sounds like the patient has benefited from support thus far. A TCA that worked in the past might not be a good choice for him now because of potential cardiac, sedating, and cognitive clouding side effects, even though he had a favorable response to it years ago. In addition, urinary difficulty from an enlarged prostate might be exacerbated by a TCA. The patient's arrhythmia makes the use of a psychostimulant less of a satisfactory medication choice. But there are SSRIs or SNRIs that the prescriber can consider that the patient might tolerate, such as sertraline, escitalopram, venlafaxine, or duloxetine. The prescriber can start a low dose of an antidepressant, and you can reinforce the need to take the medication daily and that it could take approximately a month to start seeing the benefits.

Q: The previously mentioned 79-year-old patient has been on the antidepressant for 8 weeks and the depressive symptoms are unrelenting. Is a change in the dose or the medication warranted?

A: Most likely increasing the dose of the antidepressant is reasonable now if the patient has been tolerating the medication without significant side effects. Encouraging behavioral activation is vital, as well as checking to see if there are concurrent symptoms that can be alleviated (i.e., insomnia, anxiety, pain, or severe fatigue, which may be addressed with hypnotics, anxiolytics, or pain medications) until there is relief of the depression.

NOTES

1. See https://www.nimh.nih.gov/health/statistics/major-depression.shtml and https://adaa.org/about-adaa/press-room/facts-statistics.
2. Institute of Medicine. 2008. *Cancer care for the whole patient: Meeting psychosocial health needs.* NE Adler and AEK Page, eds. Washington, DC: National Academies Press.
3. Simon GE, Stewart C, Beck A, et al. National prevalence of receipt of antidepressant prescriptions by persons without a psychiatric diagnosis. *Psychiatr Serv.* 2014; 65(7): 944–946.

Chapter 2

Anxiolytic (Antianxiety) Medications

INTRODUCTION

People with cancer develop anxiety for many reasons, including the stress of a new cancer diagnosis, complications of cancer treatment, changes in body image, fear of recurrence after treatment, dealing with recurrence or progression of their cancer after treatment, or finding out that there is no further active treatment for the cancer. Anxiety can arise from the illness experience or as an exacerbation of a pre-existing anxiety disorder. Anxiety in cancer is common and understandable, but it is not necessarily predictable, tolerable, or inevitable. As discussed with regard to depression, anxiety does not come neatly packaged as a psychiatric diagnosis ready to treat. One size does not fit all.

Anxiety affects 40 million Americans, approximately 18.1% of the population.[1] Anxiety is as common among older adults as among the young. Women are twice as likely as men to be affected by generalized anxiety disorder and panic disorder.

AVOIDING THE POTHOLES OF SUBOPTIMAL ANXIETY DIAGNOSIS IN CANCER PATIENTS

Hearing about anxiety in a person with cancer may sound normal and seem self-evident. But patients do not come into one's office packaged with a diagnosis because there are many psychiatric and medical diagnoses that can encompass anxiety symptoms (Box 2.1). Although there are many overlaps, the individual contexts of people's lives, histories, psychiatric backgrounds, and status of their cancer combine to contribute to an individual's risk of anxiety.

Box 2.1 DOES ANXIETY IN CANCER PATIENTS COME
PACKAGED AS A DIAGNOSIS?

Anxiety-Related Diagnoses

- Acute stress disorder
- Adjustment disorder with anxious/mixed features—*specific stressor*
- Anxiety disorder due to a general medical condition
- Substance-induced anxiety disorders
- Generalized anxiety disorder (6 months)
- Obsessive–compulsive disorder
- Panic disorder (four or more panic episodes in the past 6 months)
- Post-traumatic stress disorder
- Specific phobias (e.g., needle phobia or claustrophobia)
- Social anxiety

CONSIDER RISK FACTORS FOR ANXIETY SYNDROMES IN CANCER PATIENTS

As with depression, it is important to clarify psychiatric and family history for patients presenting in your office with complaints of anxiety. People with histories of anxiety or traumatic experiences are more at risk for anxiety when cancer comes into their lives. Understanding how they dealt with challenges earlier in their lives will likely give clues as to what might work now. A history of substance use or abuse may complicate getting a prescription for a minor tranquilizer from many prescribers. As with diagnosing depression, medical causes of anxiety must be considered, including uncontrolled pain; electrolyte disturbances such as hypocalcemia; endocrine anomalies such as hyperthyroidism; and medication triggers such as antinausea medication that can precipitate restlessness, or steroids that can induce a sense of frenzy, edginess, or irritability.

In this chapter, we follow the case of Jim to help understand all the potential nuances related to working with and treating cancer patients with anxiety. Toward the end of the chapter, we review the cases of Jenna, Pete, and Marie as other examples related to treating anxiety.

INTRODUCING: JIM

Jim, a 33-year-old single man with testicular cancer, just completed chemotherapy in which nausea was persistent for a few months. He was referred to you for supportive therapy. He is

---

taking antiemetics (prochlorperazine a few times every day and ondansetron as needed) and says he had been taking lorazepam. He was scheduled for retroperitoneal lymph node dissection (RPLND) for the following month and was referred to you for psychotherapy to help with coping and anxiety. Although he has completed chemotherapy, Jim continues to have nausea, and the oncologist is concerned this symptom may be more psychosomatic than physical.

While inquiring about Jim's personal and family psychiatric history, as well as the timing of his symptoms, you find out that Jim never saw a therapist or psychiatrist until recently. He saw a social worker briefly during his chemotherapy.

Jim's mother has a history of general anxiety and has been taking citalopram 20 mg daily for 15 years. Jim is not sure if his mother has ever had panic attacks.

ALGORITHM FOR DIAGNOSING SYNDROME OF ANXIETY THAT MAY REQUIRE PSYCHOTROPIC MEDICATION IN CANCER PATIENTS

Recent stressors (i.e., diagnosis, recurrence, or hearing about the need for more treatment or that there is no more active or effective treatment available)

+

Worrying, ruminating, increased irritability, or arguing

±

Physical symptoms of anxiety (i.e., pacing, palpitations, gastric/
urinary hyperactivity not related to medical issues, the
feeling of a knot in the pit of the stomach, chest discomfort,
dry mouth, shortness of breath, sweating, and a sense of
impending doom)

+

These symptoms are interfering with enjoying or managing
life, interrupting sleep, or interfering with handling medical
issues even when addressed with psychotherapy

=

*Anxiety syndrome that warrants consideration of psychotropic
medication*

Start to build an inclusive list of potential syndromes in your mind
(a differential diagnosis):

1. Jim may have an adjustment reaction to having a cancer diagnosis, and now that he has completed chemotherapy, he has
   a chance to process that information and the emotions that
   accompany it. Psychotherapy may be indicated.
2. Hearing that he needs more treatment, the RPLND, and
   is beginning to understand the potential consequences of
   that treatment can bring on anticipatory anxiety, which
   may be addressed by techniques such as cognitive–
   behavioral therapy or acceptance and commitment
   psychotherapy.
3. Many patients think they are at the end of the cancer road
   when completing a treatment and become overwhelmed
   after finding out they require further treatment. If there is
   any sense of traumatization from the initial diagnosis and

treatment, one can consider an acute or post-traumatic stress reaction. Various forms of psychotherapy may be helpful.

4. Family history can be enlightening. It could be helpful to find out whether Jim's mother had panic diforder in addition to general anxiety because this diagnosis is often strongly genetically linked or familially transmitted. If Jim's mother did have panic disorder, it is then beneficial to find out whether she was treated successfully with medication because there are indications that medications that work well for biological relatives will often also work well for the identified patient.

5. Physical symptoms have lingered beyond Jim's initial treatment. He continues to have nausea and is on an antiemetic known to cause anxiety and akathisia (prochlorperazine). Akathisia is a condition of agitation, distress, or restlessness that is often a side effect of a medication such as an antipsychotic medication or prochlorperazine or metoclopramide, which are used to relieve nausea. If Jim has akathisia, he might be best served by a change in his antiemetic regimen as well getting a benzodiazepine or propranolol to relieve his symptoms. Furthermore, because he had been on lorazepam in the recent past, you may want to consider whether he could be in withdrawal.

Jim has not been sleeping well for the previous few weeks after hearing about the need for RPLND. Since his testicular cancer was diagnosed, he knew RPLND was a possibility, but he never seriously considered it because it was not on his immediate radar screen. He has been ruminating about losing erections and not being able to ejaculate properly. He smoked marijuana occasionally for many years to help with sleep but stopped after he was diagnosed with cancer because he read on the internet that marijuana could contribute to testicular cancer.

Expanding the list of possible causes of Jim's anxiety:

1. Jim has heard about and read on the internet about potential complications of his upcoming surgery, some of which are accurate, and some are not. These are understandable reactions that may arise in a young man with cancer, who has not begun his "adult life" yet. He is not in a committed relationship currently and could benefit from discussing these issues. Psychotherapy, psychoeducation with understandable, accurate, and relevant information, and possible relaxation techniques may be helpful. He may also find it helpful to speak with his urologist again to obtain accurate information about his procedure and the relevant consequences for him, particularly regarding erections and sexual functioning.

2. It will be important to clarify how much marijuana Jim has smoked. He may have a long-standing sleep and/ or anxiety disorder that was never addressed that he was self-medicating. Although these issues precede the cancer diagnosis, if not addressed, they may impact Jim's ability to get through treatment with the least amount of distress. It could be helpful to encourage Jim to speak with his oncology team about his concerns and guilt that marijuana caused his testicular cancer so he could get accurate information that may be relevant to his circumstances.

Jim notes occasional shortness of breath, dry mouth, difficulty swallowing, and palpitations when he gets nervous as he lays in bed at night. Although he used to jog regularly, he has been afraid to exercise because of his shortness of breath.

Jim is showing possible signs of panic attacks with palpitations, dry mouth, and shortness of breath. Boxes 2.2 and 2.3 highlight

---

Box 2.2 QUESTIONS TO ASK ABOUT THE CONTEXT OF
ANXIETY IN PEOPLE WITH CANCER

Is the patient worrying about recurrence of the cancer after treatment?

Is the patient highly concerned about upcoming tests or the results of those tests (some call this *scanxiety*)?

Is the patient paradoxically anxious at the *end* of treatment?

    Feeling isolated by not being seen as often by doctor, nurses?

    Feeling a loss of protection by no longer actively treating the cancer?

Does the patient have less confidence about the future?

    Will the cancer return? When?

    Anniversaries (of diagnosis, birthdays, etc.)

Did the patient just get news about the recurrence of the cancer?

Did the patient just hear there is no more active treatment for their cancer?

Is the patient getting shortness of breath, palpitations, or a knot in the pit of their stomach?

Box 2.3 ADDITIONAL QUESTIONS TO HELP ASSESS GENERAL
ANXIETY VERSUS PANIC ATTACKS

General Anxiety Symptoms

Do the symptoms occur at certain times during the day or
are they there most of the day and/or night?

Are there possible stimuli or triggers? What are they?

Does Jim just have difficulty falling asleep or staying asleep too?

Is Jim ruminating or obsessing, going through endless worry
loops?

How often does Jim get up to urinate at night?

Does Jim get back to sleep soon after awakening?

Panic

Does Jim report physical signs of anxiety or does he mostly
fret and worry?

Palpitations or chest heaviness?

Shortness of breath?

Dry mouth or difficulty swallowing?

The feeling of a knot in the pit of his stomach?

Shakiness or tremors?

A sense of restlessness, difficulty sitting still, pacing, or dizziness?

A sense of impending doom, death, or feeling "I'm going crazy!"?

If Jim wakes up with panic, how long does it take to get back
to sleep?

Bottom line: If Jim's symptoms interfere with his ability to
carry out activities or enjoy life, even with psychotherapy, a
medication may be needed for his anxiety.

questions that help navigate the complexity of coexisting panic symptoms, generalized worry, and other overlapping physical symptoms in the context of cancer treatment, in addition to the difficulty practitioners have in teasing out a diagnosis that will lead to a clear treatment road map.

Whether the symptoms of anxiety will tip a non-prescriber to suggest a referral to a prescriber for a medication to address anxiety may depend on the answers to the following questions:

1. Can you clarify Jim's symptoms in more detailed terms, including getting a better sense of the timing of onset and duration of Jim's symptoms?
2. How often was Jim taking lorazepam and for how long? When did he stop taking it? How much was he taking each time?
3. Was Jim taking lorazepam more often for nausea, anxiety, sleep, or all three?
4. Can you find out whether there is a temporal relationship between Jim's anxiety symptoms and smoking marijuana? What other medications or substances has Jim been using, including over-the-counter diphenhydramine for sleep, caffeine, etc.?
5. Do Jim's symptoms ever occur during the day, or do they occur mostly at night?
6. Are Jim's anxiety and worry constant, or do they occur in spurts or waves?
7. Can Jim identify possible stimuli or triggers for his anxiety?
8. Does Jim always get palpitations, dry mouth, and shortness of breath when these episodes occur?
9. Can Jim describe what he is doing or thinking about before the symptoms arise?

10. Is there anything Jim does that relieves the discomfort?

11. Are there symptoms that could be identified as bodily or position-specific (i.e., do they only occur when lying down, or upon rising or standing up)?

Given Jim's recent chemotherapy, the physical symptoms need to be clarified by his primary medical doctor, oncologist, or urologist to ensure they are not medical in origin.

You begin to teach Jim relaxation and breathing exercises. Furthermore, you can explore cognitive reframing (i.e., consideration of alternative yet plausible perspectives or scenarios) for his catastrophic (e.g., worst-case) scenario and/or forecasting (e.g., predicting based on fear or subjective concerns rather than objective data) about possible complications that could arise from his upcoming surgery. Jim, however, has difficulty sitting still as he tries to follow your directions. After closing his eyes for 20 seconds, he opens them and says this is a waste of time. Further questioning will help you get a better picture of the recent past that might explain the present:

If Jim was taking lorazepam regularly, was it stopped abruptly? Could this be withdrawal or are you seeing untreated anxiety?

Even if you do not see obvious restlessness, ask Jim if he feels a need to pace or keep his limbs moving. If he does, could this be akathisia? This is often described by patients as "I feel like I am jumping out of my skin."

Jim notes that he had been taking lorazepam for nausea during chemotherapy and stopped it abruptly when he stopped chemotherapy. But he is still taking prochlorperazine to prevent nausea. You note that he could be in withdrawal from lorazepam and will need help from his oncologist or a psychiatrist to restart lorazepam, a benzodiazepine, briefly, as the other antiemetic does not prevent benzodiazepine withdrawal. Jim will then need to taper off lorazepam when he is ready to stop it in order to avoid further withdrawal symptoms.

Withdrawal or akathisia will make sitting through a psychotherapy session quite challenging. It would be quite difficult to review sleep hygiene strategies or teach a relaxation exercise while someone is so agitated or fidgety.

Jim has anxiety symptoms of worry and restlessness, as well as panic indicators that include palpitations, sweating, butterflies in the abdomen, dry or tight throat, and even dizziness.

At this point, you tell Jim that you and he should check with his oncologist about a physical side effect of his antiemetic that could also cause his restlessness, called akathisia. This may need to be addressed before you can address his symptoms with psychotherapy. You also support Jim getting medication treatment for possible panic symptoms for a brief period while he learns from you the therapeutic tools to keep his anxiety manageable.

People tend to experience anxiety in unique ways, even though they might react similarly to specific anxiety-provoking situations. Therefore, in order to determine the best treatment for anxiety, it is important to consider the components of the etiology and the timing of the appearance of symptoms, which may be understood by acuteness of onset; prior history of anxiety; relationship to stressors, situations, or other variables; as well as the intensity of symptoms. Initially, however, if the symptoms are more physical in nature, they should be assessed medically rather than assuming that they are merely related to anxiety. Patients with panic symptoms can go through one or more medical workups, often in emergency rooms or urgent care settings, for cardiac, pulmonary, or gastric complaints before a decision is made to treat psychiatrically.

CHALLENGES OF TREATING ANXIETY IN PEOPLE WITH CANCER

If anxiety interferes with a person's ability to get on with or enjoy their life as they are living with cancer during or after cancer treatment, and psychotherapy, distraction, or relaxation techniques are inadequate to sufficiently lessen the anxiety, a medication intervention can be useful. Significant interruptions in concentration at work, school, or home because of anxiety symptoms may warrant an evaluation for a psychotropic medication. It is not good enough to say, "Well, Jim has cancer; of course, he's anxious. Wouldn't anyone be anxious?"

Table 2.1 highlights the importance of not just seeing the psychological manifestations of an anxious symptom or syndrome but also understanding the possible biologic underpinning of those symptoms. Anxiety, worry, panic, and restlessness can be physiological reactions to cancer treatment or to other medications and not merely reactions to stressful situations, as discussed previously with regard to depression. It is important to also note the situational context of the development or surge of anxiety.

Table 2.1 Beware Medical Look-Alike Causes of Anxiety—They Need Addressing

Metabolic	Medication Induced	Other	Substances
Hypoxia	Corticosteroids	Pain	Intoxication
Delirium	Dexamethasone	Balance problems	Withdrawal
Sepsis	Prednisone	Sensory losses	
Bleeding	Antiemetics (akathisia)	Endocrine anomalies	
Pulmonary embolus	Bronchodilators		
Hypocalcemia	Hormonal agents		

ARE THERE ANY LABORATORY TESTS THAT MIGHT HELP CLARIFY AN ANXIETY DIAGNOSIS?

Primary care doctors, nurse practitioners, and oncology teams may consider obtaining the following labs to identify abnormalities that can cause anxiety:

Vital signs to include orthostatic blood pressure
Thyroid function tests (hyperthyroidism can make people feel anxious and restless)
Urinary analysis/culture (urinary tract infections can make patients uncomfortable)

Electrolyte assessment (hypocalcemia—low calcium—can
    cause anxiety and restlessness)
Complete blood count for possible anemia
Chest X-ray for causes of shortness of breath
Electrocardiogram for possible arrhythmias

It is important to review psychological responses of worry and panic to stressful situations as well as side effects of cancer or cancer treatments that may appear to be psychological in real time but which are medical in cause and evolution. The latter will require a medical response or intervention. Higher anxiety intensity can impair a patient's ability to make treatment decisions, impact compliance with treatment, and contribute to suboptimal functioning. Consequently, inadequately recognized and treated anxiety, as well as other psychiatric disorders such as depression and delirium, can inadvertently prolong hospital stays beyond the obvious medical necessity. Pharmacologic treatment for cancer-related anxiety, alone or in combination with psychotherapy, can reduce emotional distress and facilitate cancer treatment.

Tips for Communicating with the Prescriber—
Two Scenarios

You decide to make the referral to the oncologist, general practitioner, or psychiatrist and continue to provide support to the patient. The discussion with the prescriber may go as follows:

I have been following Jim for anxiety for the last few weeks. He has worries about his cancer and treatment, but I have found that his anxiety has characteristics of panic disorder.

SCENARIO A

I am concerned that Jim was taking lorazepam for nausea and occasionally for anxiety for over a month but stopped a week ago when he ran out of it. He did not call for a refill because his chemotherapy was completed, but he was taking it up to three times a day for many weeks, and is still taking prochlorperazine for nausea. Do you think this could be withdrawal in addition to his understandable worries? [The prescriber may order a prescription for lorazepam stat or the patient will be asked to go to the emergency room because one of the more dangerous complications of benzodiazepine withdrawal, although rare, is seizures, which could be life-threatening.]

SCENARIO B

Jim has difficulty sitting still, feeling a need to pace. He says he feels like he is "jumping out of my skin." I wonder if this could be akathisia related to the prochlorperazine [or metoclopramide] he has been taking for nausea recently. As you know, this side effect is quite uncomfortable and has even led some patients to think about suicide, as they cannot tolerate an unbearable physical sensation like this, especially if they do not understand why it is happening.

ASK, BECAUSE THEY MAY NOT TELL

Jim sees his oncologist, who tells him that akathisia can be treated with either a benzodiazepine or a β-blocker, like propranolol. The oncologist takes him off of prochlorperazine and expects that Jim's nausea will continue to improve during the next month. He prescribes lorazepam, which helps both the anxiety and nausea, as well as possible withdrawal symptoms.

Jim returns to see you a week later and says he is feeling somewhat better since he stopped taking prochlorperazine and restarted the lorazepam. He is less restless. You wonder if he is feeling better because akathisia was treated or if he had been in benzodiazepine withdrawal that is now getting treated. But it doesn't really matter. He is better.

However, he tells you that he is afraid to take lorazepam at night because he read in the package insert that it could cause trouble breathing. The oncologist did not find physiological concerns for shortness of breath (i.e., no pneumonia, no pulmonary embolus, and no other signs of infection). There were also no signs of cardiac rhythm abnormalities.

If you only spoke with the oncologist and did not ask Jim about his compliance with his medications, you might not hear about Jim's fears of taking lorazepam. Additional questions for enquiry are listed in Box 2.4.

Box 2.4 ADDITIONAL QUESTIONS TO CLARIFY NIGHT
ANXIETY AND SLEEP DISTURBANCE

Does Jim have trouble falling asleep?

Does he wake up in the middle of the night and then have
trouble getting back to sleep?

Does Jim lie awake as his mind ruminates about various
issues?

Can Jim clarify whether his awakenings in the middle of the
night are related to anxiety? Or are the awakenings related to
physical causes, such as needing to urinate or having pain?

Urinary frequency or pain can be exacerbated by anxiety
or medical reasons. If there are any questions related to urinary
habits, patients should check with their urologist or primary care
doctor just to make sure.

You remind Jim that his oncologist did not find any problems
and that he had taken lorazepam for several weeks without shortness
of breath. Slowly you encourage behavioral activation (walking) so
Jim can gain confidence in his cardiopulmonary systems again. You
can discuss with Jim that people often experience anxiety at night
when there are few other distractions. You ask him to describe some
of his anxious thoughts.

When you see Jim the following week, he has calmed down significantly. He is taking lorazepam regularly as recommended and has

started tapering it very slowly. When you try to discuss his fears about retrograde ejaculation, he gets sweaty and says he is not sure he can go through with the surgery. He feels the palpitations starting again and says he is having trouble catching his breath.

You are glad Jim got cardiac clearance from his treatment team. You are now concerned about the possibility of panic disorder, given his physiological anxiety responses of sweating, shortness of breath, palpitations, and dry mouth with difficulty swallowing. He answers affirmatively to your question about whether he feels a knot in the pit of stomach. You note mild tremulousness and ask about dizziness and restlessness. He says he might feel more comfortable if he paces in your office to relieve his angst, and asks if that is OK, because he does not think he can sit through the rest of the session.

Box 2.5   THE DIFFERENTIAL DIAGNOSIS FOR JIM AT THIS POINT

- Adjustment disorder with anxious features**
- Anxiety disorder due to another medical condition**
- Panic disorder**
- Generalized anxiety disorder*
- Substance/medication withdrawal **
- Intoxication/substance use**
- Post-traumatic stress disorder*
- Obsessive–compulsive disorder***

Key

* The practitioner should consider more specific diagnostic possibilities with more data, time, and increased history.

** These anxiety diagnoses are either likely, or already proven for Jim.

*** This diagnosis is usually made by obtaining more history.

As with depression, it is useful not only to have a differential diagnosis in mind, as noted in Box 2.5, but also to hone it as you gather more information. Keep in mind that anxiety can have multiple etiologies even in the same patient at different times. With a refined idea of origins of anxiety, you have a better sense of what you need to focus on, what needs to be addressed by Jim's medical team, and what may need to be directed to a psychiatrist. A discussion with the prescriber about these developments leads to a decision to slow down the taper of lorazepam.

UNDERSTANDING THE STRATEGIES OF THE PSYCHO-ONCOLOGY MEDICATION PRESCRIBER

Overview of Antianxiety Medications

There are many medications to treat the symptoms of anxiety, but not all are ideal in people with cancer. If the symptoms remain once any potential sources of the symptoms are decreased or removed, and the psychological tools used in psychotherapy are either not helpful or not easily integrated during an anxiety crisis, benzodiazepines are the drug of choice for immediate, short-term relief of anxiety symptoms, including the situational distress and fear that arise before or during medical procedures such as magnetic resonance imaging (MRI) scans or biopsies. These medications are usually well-tolerated, safe, and effective for use in cancer patients. In addition, benzodiazepines relieve panic attacks, insomnia, chemotherapy-related nausea, and medication-induced akathisia. Antidepressants are helpful for longer term relief and prevention of generalized anxiety and panic symptoms. Other non-benzodiazepines, such as atypical antipsychotics, antihistamines, buspirone, and propranolol, can be used for various anxiety or panic symptoms depending on the situation and if the prescriber wants to avoid benzodiazepines, although they may not be as effective.

THE MEDESCORT GUIDE FOR ANXIOLYTICS

Medication Options for Anxiety That the Prescriber May Consider

Benzodiazepines—minor tranquilizers as primary treatment for anxiety, panic or akathisia, as well as certain substance withdrawal

Alprazolam (Xanax)

Lorazepam (Ativan)

Diazepam (Valium)

Clonazepam (Klonopin)

Non-benzodiazepine anxiolytics (as longer term anxiety prevention)

Buspirone

Antidepressants—selective serotonin reuptake inhibitors (SSRIs)/serotonin norepinephrine reuptake inhibitors (SNRIs)

Citalopram (Celexa)

Escitalopram (Lexapro)

Fluoxetine (Prozac)

Paroxetine (Paxil)

Sertraline (Zoloft)

Vortioxetine (Trintellix)

Venlafaxine (Effexor)

Desvenlafaxine (Pristiq)

Mirtazapine (Remeron)

Duloxetine (Cymbalta)

Antipsychotics—major tranquilizers

Olanzapine (Zyprexa)

Quetiapine (Seroquel)

Loxapine (Loxitane)

Antihistaminic medications

Hydroxyzine (Vistaril)

Diphenhydramine (Benadryl)

Antiseizure medications

Gabapentin (Neurontin)

Pregabalin (Lyrica)

Propranolol—a β-blocker that has been found to be helpful
for akathisia, performance anxiety, and essential tremors

A patient such as Jim who has an acute panic attack needs relief fast.
He cannot wait hours, let alone weeks, for an antidepressant to have
an effect. Benzodiazepines work quickly. Although antidepressants
take weeks to have a beneficial effect for anxiety and depression,
they are helpful to prevent further panic attacks and, therefore the
subsequent fear of having another panic attack in the future.

MEDICATION TREATMENT CONSIDERATIONS
FOR PANIC DISORDER BY THE PRESCRIBER

Benzodiazepine

Which is the best to use and for how long?

Which is the best to avoid?

Antidepressant

Which is the best to use and for how long?

Which is the best to avoid?

It is important to understand how different anxiolytic medications work and why one class of medication may be preferred for the treatment of a specific type of anxiety in a specific situation. You will learn to distinguish drug dependence, drug tolerance, and drug addiction—terms that are often mistakenly confused even by medical professionals, which can lead to inadequate care. With this knowledge, you will be able to alleviate the angst about patients with cancer taking medications that might significantly improve emotional and physical quality of life.

BENZODIAZEPINES

How Benzodiazepines Work

We think it is important for the non-prescribing clinician, and the patients who may have benzodiazepines prescribed, to know how these medications work. Useful information can prompt improved adherence and safety. Benzodiazepines taken orally are absorbed in the stomach and small intestine, distributed through the bloodstream through the body, and preferentially accumulate in lipid-rich areas. They cross the blood–brain barrier, acting in parts of the brain that modulate anxiety, stress, sleep, seizures, and other functions. They are eventually metabolized by the liver; many have active metabolites that require further breakdown, whereas some are not further changed (i.e., lorazepam, oxazepam, and temazepam) and have more predictability in how long they stay in the body before excretion in the urine. A number of brain areas are involved in controlling anxiety, including the locus ceruleus, the amygdala, the limbic system, and the hippocampus. Neurotransmitter networks that appear to be involved in modulating anxiety in the brain include, but are not limited to, γ-aminobutyric acid (GABA), serotonin, opioid peptides, cannabinoids, oxytocin, neuropeptide Y, oxytocin, and corticotropin-releasing hormone.

Benzodiazepines enhance the effectiveness of GABA receptors to allow GABA transmitters to have an inhibitory or calming effect. If the brain is overwhelmed in an excitatory state of anxiety (or sleeplessness), it needs to get some of that hyperarousal dissolved. The natural inhibitory receptors in the amygdala, a part of the limbic system of the brain, are in charge of that calming function. For GABA receptors located in the musculoskeletal system, benzodiazepine medications help provide muscle relaxation. In the brain, they decrease anxiety and enhance sleep. When people experience high anxiety or panic, those natural receptors often cannot produce enough inhibition or relief. A benzodiazepine interacts with the proper part of the GABA receptor, leading to enhanced transmission that promotes inhibitory effects, allowing more relief from anxiety, panic, or sleeplessness.

However, benzodiazepines scare many patients. They are thought to be *drugs*. The perception that they can be abused leads to many incorrect ideas when they are recommended by health care

---

Box 2.6 MYTHS THAT KEEP PATIENTS FROM TAKING BENZODIAZEPINES

Address These Topics with Patients
  "I will become addicted."
  "I won't have control over what I say or do."
  "I heard you can get dementia from these tranquilizers."
  "I heard these medications treat seizures. Why should I take them for anxiety?"

---

providers. These myths are barriers to using medications that might be able to improve quality of life (Box 2.6).

There is some reality to these myths; however, patients need to understand the facts about these medications as best we know them. First, as explained later, addiction can be a consequence of using these medications when taken inappropriately. Many over-the-counter substances can cause addiction, including alcohol, cigarettes, and even sleep or cold medications that contain diphenhydramine or alcohol. Some patients with histories of addiction to these substances may be more at risk for addiction with benzodiazepines. When benzodiazepines are prescribed in the cancer setting for brief periods of time, with responsible monitoring, they do not usually lead to addiction.

It is important to note that benzodiazepines, like alcohol, should not be taken if one must drive a car or use heavy machinery. Benzodiazepines, as with alcohol, can cause sedation, unsteadiness, and poor coordination. Although rare, some people can become disinhibited. They may cry more easily, become irritated with little provocation, or feel cloudy. Severe effects can include memory loss, mood swings, erratic behavior, and paradoxical anxiety.

A few studies have found an association between benzodiazepine use and dementia. However, these studies were not designed to assess causality, so it is not clear what variables, other than the benzodiazepines, could be responsible for causing dementia. Findings such as this have also been reported in recent studies that have found an association between antidepressants and dementia. Causality has not been proven. Indeed, studies show that depression in older people can also lead to dementia. What a dilemma: Suffer with depression or take a medication to relieve it but that might have long-term unwanted consequences. Although these studies are concerning, we do not believe they should impact treating someone with cancer who may be going through arduous cancer treatment and has significant anxiety or depression related to that.

Why We Use Benzodiazepines for People with Cancer

Benzodiazepines are probably the most prescribed antianxiety medications since the discovery of chlordiazepoxide in the 1950s and the introduction of chlordiazepoxide and diazepam in the 1960s as alternatives to barbiturates. They are prescribed as controlled substances because of their potential for misuse and subsequent harm. Although these medications can be addictive, their potential benefits generally outweigh their risks in cancer patients.

Benzodiazepines are important medications to address worry and panic attacks in cancer patients. It was initially hoped that these sedative medications would have an improved side effect profile, including less respiratory depression, which was a major limitation of barbiturates, the primary tranquilizing medications at the time.

We do not discuss all the medications in the benzodiazepine class. We review only the ones that psycho-oncologists have found most helpful in people with cancer. Because these medications cause drowsiness, they are also used to treat insomnia; however, like most other sleep medications, their use is not recommended for extended periods of time, given the problems regarding dependence and tolerance. In addition, without occasional trials of medication-free periods to see if sleep–wake cycles have had a chance to normalize, a sleep medication that gets started may never be discontinued. Beyond a maximum suggested dose, or ceiling, a patient can more often anticipate side effects rather than benefits. Because of the potential for addiction, treatment should be monitored in people with histories of substance use disorders, whether from substances such as alcohol, or medications such as barbiturates, cocaine, or opiates. We discuss sleep medications in Chapter 4. It is important to note, however, that most medications that can cause enough drowsiness to facilitate sleep can cause unsteadiness or forgetfulness. Muscle coordination or balance can be compromised, which can lead to falls if a patient awakens in the middle of the night and tries to walk. Night lights can be a useful safety recommendation for these patients by facilitating faster reorientation. Recall that benzodiazepines work in the same area of the brain, and on the same neurotransmitters, as alcohol. They are cleaner pharmacologically than alcohol, meaning they have more precise and consistent brain targets. but they can have similar negative effects, including balance and concentration problems—although they do not taste as good (or bad depending on your taste buds). So instead of experiencing a calming result, a patient can become unexpectedly more anxious, irritable, disinhibited, or even confused.

MAKING BENZODIAZEPINES MULTITASK: THE BENEFITS MAY OFFER TWOFERS (OR MORE)

Benzodiazepines have been used as hypnotics to initiate grogginess and sleep. Sometimes difficulty sleeping is related to anxiety, so giving an anxious person a non-benzodiazepine hypnotic such as zolpidem does not necessarily fix the problem, even temporarily. A benzodiazepine can relieve a panic attack, more general worry and anxiety, and induce sleep. Benzodiazepines can also relieve nausea. Some benzodiazepines can relax muscles and in the short term can help with minor muscles spasms or strains (Box 2.7).

Box 2.7 BENZO ADVANTAGES: THE POSITIVE EFFECTS OF
BENZODIAZEPINES

- Can relieve worry
- Can decrease restlessness/pacing
- Can relieve panic symptoms
  - Palpitations, diaphoresis, and shortness of breath
- Can initiate sleep and combat insomnia—best if not used regularly for long periods of time to avoid dependence and tolerance
- Can improve irritability
- Can lessen chemotherapy-related nausea
- Can decrease anticipatory anxiety prior to medical procedures or while waiting for test results
  - Patients should inform their doctors if they take a benzodiazepine before a medical procedure.
- Can decrease fear of flying, which can be helpful when patients can take a break from cancer treatment for a vacation
- Can treat seizures
- Can enhance muscle relaxation

POTENTIAL POTHOLES OF BENZODIAZEPINE TREATMENT

Common Side Effects of Benzodiazepines

In addition to relaxation and sleep, the inhibitory effects of benzodiazepines can also cause sedation, problems concentrating, forgetfulness, dizziness, and muscle relaxation, which in excess can

Box 2.8 BENZODIAZEPINE SIDE EFFECTS

- Drowsiness
- Respiratory depression
- Impaired coordination
- Memory loss
- Paradoxical anxiety and agitation rather than calming effect
- Dependence, tolerance, and addiction

lead to problems with ambulation, driving, focusing, and working. Individually or combined, these side effects make falls and other accidents more likely in vulnerable populations (Box 2.8).

SAFETY: INFORM PATIENTS ABOUT THESE REACTIONS AND POTENTIAL CONTRAINDICATIONS

The side effects of forgetfulness, confusion, falls, and habituation or "getting hooked" on benzodiazepines make patients and practitioners fearful of these prescriptions. Complications occur more readily if a patient is consuming alcohol or taking other central nervous system depressant medications while taking benzodiazepines. If the patient is taking more than one medication in the benzodiazepine class even for different purposes (e.g., alprazolam for anxiety or panic attacks, lorazepam for nausea, and temazepam for sleep), they can develop an accumulative, compounded problem.

A person can be charged with driving while intoxicated or driving under the influence for driving after using either alcohol or a benzodiazepine. People who are in the excitatory state of alcohol withdrawal after stopping prolonged use of alcohol abruptly can benefit from benzodiazepines to quiet the withdrawal symptoms that at worst can include seizures. However, this is also why recovering alcoholics are directed to avoid routine benzodiazepine use because these can reignite cravings for alcohol. It is important to inform patients about these and other potential negative effects of benzodiazepines before they develop these problems. Use of alcohol and benzodiazepines simultaneously can cause respiratory depression, or slowing, and death. People who have histories of substance abuse can still be prescribed benzodiazepines when they are going through cancer treatment; however, prescribers need to keep close watch and monitor usage.

Prescribers will be alert to which patients should avoid benzodiazepines or, for those who are prescribed the medications, to advise using extreme caution. Aging patients and those with liver disease are less likely to be prescribed benzodiazepines; if they are prescribed one, it is best to use one that bypasses liver metabolism and is broken down in the kidneys. On the other hand, benzodiazepines such as lorazepam and oxazepam, which are cleared primarily by the kidneys, are contraindicated in patients who have a history of kidney disease. Patients with cognitive disorders or dementia should not be prescribed medications such as benzodiazepines that are likely to fog thinking even more. Unless a patient with high, regular intake of alcohol is currently receiving a benzodiazepine for detoxification to prevent withdrawal, they should not get a standing dose of a benzodiazepine. Elderly people who may be at risk of falls should probably not take benzodiazepines, even if they are cognitively intact. Prescribers will be alert to patients who are taking other medications that can interact with benzodiazepines, including antiseizure medications and other central nervous system depressants such as opioids. Benzodiazepines can depress respirations, so patients may have more compromised breathing with a benzodiazepine. A patient who is anxious because they have shortness of breath is not likely to do well with a benzodiazepine because it may make the whole cascade of breathing problems that is the cause of the anxiety even worse. Some patients with sleep apnea are prescribed benzodiazepines to decrease their angst about wearing a mask for their nighttime airway pressure machines; however, these medications can also cause problems for these patients because their respiratory drive may be impaired.

There are few data about use of benzodiazepines in pregnant women with cancer. Caution should be taken, with care to use shorter to intermediate-acting benzodiazepines and to be aware of passing depressant effects to infants through breast-feeding. Consultation with a psychiatrist who specializes in neonatal and postnatal care may bring calm to all concerned.

Box 2.9 shows which patients are more at risk of not tolerating benzodiazepines and who should be forewarned and perhaps not be given benzodiazepine prescriptions.

Box 2.9 VULNERABLE PATIENTS WHO MAY NOT TOLERATE
BENZODIAZEPINES WELL

- People aged 70 years or older or who are frail
- Those with a history of cognitive disorder or deficits
- Those with impaired liver or kidney function
- Patients with impaired balance or ambulation
- Patients with compromised breathing
- Those with a history of substance addiction or abuse or current use of substances (especially alcohol, benzodiazepines, or opioids)
- Pregnant women

TAKING ANXIETY MEDICATIONS REGULARLY (OR OTHER MEDICATIONS THAT MAY BE ADDICTIVE FOR SOME) DOES NOT MAKE ONE AN ADDICT

The Importance of Distinguishing Dependence, Tolerance, and Addiction

If you and your patients do not understand the differences between dependence, tolerance, and addiction, your patients might suffer unnecessarily. This is a vital issue for patients, prescribers, and non-prescribers to clearly understand. Here, we describe the differences so you can help explain them to patients and, along with the primary prescriber, help monitor for them.

PHYSICAL DEPENDENCE

Physical dependence is likely in most, if not all, people taking a benzodiazepine daily for a prolonged period. This means that abrupt cessation after a month or more of daily use can lead to withdrawal symptoms—a physical phenomenon. Withdrawal symptoms may include anxiety, restlessness, sweating, palpitations, insomnia, and, rarely, seizures. Although seizures are rare, they are the most feared withdrawal symptom because they can be deadly. However, there is no reason for anyone to suffer dangerous withdrawal from a benzodiazepine if the dose of the medication is tapered slowly—this can take a few weeks or longer.

PHYSICAL TOLERANCE

After a few months of daily benzodiazepine treatment, some patients do not get the same "bang for the buck" and require higher doses in order to get the same amount of anxiety relief they previously got with lower doses. Although it appears to some as if these patients are addicted because they are asking for higher doses or more frequent prescriptions, this is not necessarily the case. This may be a physiological response and not a psychological, addictive phenomenon. Sometimes practitioners inadvertently treat "pseudo-addiction" and wind up in a clinical bind. They are hesitant to give more of a medication that can be addictive and that may have strict state and federal prescribing controls. However, they also do not want their patients to suffer, and their patients may need justifiably higher doses of the medication for adequate relief. This same paradox is seen with people who are treated for cancer-related pain, in part because of the fear that has been imposed about prescribing opioids for non-cancer-related pain syndromes. Prescribers need to monitor patients carefully but should avoid inadvertently contributing to more suffering in cancer patients by underprescribing antianxiety or pain medications. Reports from non-prescribing clinicians about the fidelity to proper use and the benefits received from benzodiazepines can be reassuring to all.

PSYCHOLOGICAL AND BIOCHEMICAL ADDICTION

Addiction is thought of as compulsive use of a substance despite harm:

- The substance is often used in larger amounts than is indicated.
- There is a persistent desire or there are unsuccessful efforts to reduce or control substance use.

- People with substance use disorders spend a great deal of time in activities necessary to obtain, use, or recover from the substance.
- People with substance use disorders often have problematic social, occupational, or recreational activities because of their substance use.

When considering prescribing controlled substances, prescribers fear facilitating addiction or creating a new complication in someone who already has medical problems. They are concerned about misuse of a medication that could cause harm to the patient or others. They may be concerned that patients will sell or give their medications to others. They worry that patients may overuse the medications and request more medication before the prescription is due. Prescribers are also concerned about reliable patients who live in suboptimal settings who may have their medication stolen, misused, or misdirected from its intended use and user because a family member or friend has an addiction or sells the medication on the street to make money. This is called diversion of the medication. Safety issues can be identified by frequent requests for the controlled substance (as long as pseudo-addiction and real need are also considered).

The non-prescriber may be the most important bridge between the patient and the prescriber getting on the same page to medically responsible care. Understanding the distinctions between dependence, tolerance, and addiction as well as pseudo-addiction, and your willingness and competence to educate and review these unique and sometimes misunderstood characteristics with patients, families, and sometimes the prescriber, can be the difference between feeling like a police officer and being a successful, compassionate caregiver (Box 2.10).

Box 2.10 EDUCATE PATIENTS ABOUT BENZODIAZEPINE USE,
ADDITIONAL NEED, AND MISUSE

Physical dependence: Common—develops after approximately 1 month of daily use.

Physical *tolerance*: Less common—may lead some patients to require a higher dose after a few months of daily treatment to obtain the same amount of relief they obtained previously with lower doses; can be mistaken for "pseudo-addiction".

Addiction: Least common—compulsive psychological and biochemical drug-seeking behaviors. Prescribers and non-prescribers need to be aware of diversion of medication by patients or others for non-intended purposes. Addiction can be seen with use of other substances such as opioids, sleep medications, over-the-counter medications such as antihistamines, alcohol, and other drugs of abuse, as well as behaviors such as gambling and food addictions (i.e., use or overuse despite harm).

Jim is young and has no history of cognitive, liver, or kidney function problems. Apart from his newly diagnosed testicular cancer, he is in good health. It would be helpful for the non-prescribing clinician to educate about, and reinforce the distinctions between dependence, tolerance, and addiction. Given his past use of marijuana, we also want to try to understand if Jim was self-treating a sleep or anxiety disorder with marijuana, or if there was any component related to addiction.

DRUG INTERACTIONS

As with antidepressants, benzodiazepines can interact with medications that simultaneously travel through the blood, liver, or kidneys. Online tables or charts for these interactions should be checked by prescribers. Non-prescribers who are aware of all other medications that their patients are taking may help flag potential hazards. Prescribers can decide along with the patient that a risk:benefit ratio is acceptable for the patient or situation. Prescribers should assume that patients will read about potential interactions and may want to have discussions about these issues. Non-prescribers may be asked to help patients assess their particular risk:benefit ratio.

UNDERSTANDING THE STRATEGIES OF THE PSYCHO-ONCOLOGY PRESCRIBER

How a Prescriber Thinks About Prescribing an Antianxiety Medication

The potential advantages and disadvantages of benzodiazepine medications are often determined by how quickly they work, how long their effects last, and their side effect profiles. These qualities help prescribers decide in different situations which antianxiety medication might be best tolerated and which will achieve the overall goal of treatment. Benzodiazepines that have intermediate lasting effects (i.e., alprazolam and lorazepam) relieve procedure-related worry and anticipatory anxiety, panic attacks, and medically related phobias (e.g., fear of getting injections or seeing intravenous needles; or staying in closed MRI scans for an unpredictable length of time) with less likelihood of having a prolonged hangover effect afterwards. Very short-acting benzodiazepines (e.g., oxazepam) might not last long enough to complete the entire procedure. Longer acting anxiolytics, such as clonazepam or diazepam, may help with the unpredictable timing of hospital routines and decrease the potential for rebound anxiety or end-of-dose failure sometimes seen with shorter acting benzodiazepines, although they may leave a hangover feeling after the procedure is completed.

Jim's oncologist suggested lorazepam for Jim's anxiety and nausea because it worked for him in the past. If Jim inadvertently put himself in withdrawal by stopping his medication abruptly, he will need go on a standing dose of lorazepam again to calm his system and eventually have the lorazepam tapered slowly. Lorazepam is moderately fast acting, so Jim will not wait a long time for it to help him fall asleep. If he has a panic attack at night, lorazepam will take longer than alprazolam or diazepam to have an effect. On the other hand, it may take longer for Jim to feel relief from lorazepam compared to shorter onset oxazepam, but with a less abrupt ending to its effect, also known as rebound anxiety, as seen with alprazolam. It might therefore provide a longer night's sleep and smoother anxiety control during the day. It is also possible that the onset of Jim's panic attacks coincided with the abrupt discontinuation of lorazepam. Thus, his panic symptoms may have been secondary to withdrawal symptoms. However, clinicians need to be aware that panic symptoms that begin for any reason can beget future panic symptoms, even without the same instigating propellant.

In the oncology setting, prescribers consider the following factors when choosing medications to prescribe for patients: how fast or slow it can take for a medication to work, how long the medication is likely to have an effect for a patient, potential side effects in the context of a patient's medical and psychological vulnerabilities, psychiatric history, and past experience with various antianxiety medications or substances (Box 2.11).

When patients have panic symptoms or a worrisome medical procedure must be performed, they do not want to wait weeks for

---

Box 2.11 ONSET OF ACTION: FAST IS GOOD BUT NOT
ALWAYS BETTER

Fast-Onset Anxiolytics: Relieve Panic Attacks Quickly

Treat phobic symptoms related to medical procedures (MRI scans, awaiting test results).

Relieve akathisia (restlessness) caused by other medications (older antiemetics).

Control agitation during acute manic episodes in medical settings.

Treat alcohol withdrawal.

Slower Onset of Action

Less potential for addiction.

Does not reinforce crisis-related relief.

a medication (a non-benzodiazepine) to take effect. But if they do not know when an anxiety-provoking situation will occur, a non-benzodiazepine might be just the medication to prevent escalating anxiety (Box 2.12).

A few weeks after restarting lorazepam, Jim comes to you for a therapy session. He says enthusiastically that since restarting lorazepam, his panic symptoms and sleep have improved. He is not experiencing

---

Box 2.12 THE LONG AND SHORT OF BENZODIAZEPINES

Shorter Acting Benzodiazepines (e.g., Oxazepam)

  Less chance of hangover effect
  Usually not good for a full night's sleep
  May cause rebound anxiety

Intermediate-Acting Benzodiazepines (e.g., Alprazolam, Lorazepam)

  Excellent for brief anxiety episodes
  Less chance of hangover effect
  May not be as good for a full night's sleep

Longer Acting Benzodiazepines (i.e., Clonazepam)

  Excellent for relief of more free-floating, less predictable anxiety
  Less chance for rebound anxiety breakthrough
  Better for maintaining a longer night's sleep
  Increased likelihood of "hangover effect"

---

any shortness of breath, and his nausea has subsided. However, he tells you that he wakes up feeling groggy, feeling as if his head is in a cloud. He says he has to wait a couple of hours before feeling clear enough to drive his car to his job. You reinforce his appropriate behavior, as a hangover or intoxication from a benzodiazepine can be as dangerous as from alcohol. You suggest he inform his prescriber about this hangover feeling. You discuss the possibility of Jim getting a ride to work from a co-worker until he can start to taper the lorazepam. You may also note to yourself that it is probably good that he is not taking a longer acting benzodiazepine such as clonazepam or diazepam, in case his prescribers consider those in the future.

ALPRAZOLAM (XANAX)

Alprazolam is an intermediate-acting benzodiazepine with a fast onset of action. Thus, it is best used on an as-needed basis for people who have periodic or intermittent anxiety symptoms or panic attacks. Alprazolam is not ideal for daily use for long stretches of anxiety. Another midrange-acting medication, such as lorazepam, can be used on a regular basis for 1 or 2 weeks prior to anxiety-provoking situations such as undergoing computed tomography scans, medical procedures, and receiving test results of tumor markers, blood tests, or biopsies. It is important to determine if the patient can function well without an antianxiety medication after the worrisome or crisis period has concluded, although for some patients, these periods can extend for weeks or months. Anxious patients often feel that the fate of their lives hangs in the balance of the result of an upcoming test or scan, like a magic prediction ball: "Win or lose; live or die." Alprazolam acts quickly in the body. It can bring relief for a few hours, so there is rarely a "hangover" effect that would otherwise leave patients feeling groggy or even disoriented once the panic- or anxiety-provoking situation has passed. Although alprazolam has a welcome quick onset of action, can have a rather abrupt end to its effect, causing rebound anxiety for many people. When this happens, patients feel as anxious as when they took the medication in the first place, and sometimes even more so. They rapidly feel their anxiety return, feeling much worse than just a short while before. Often, patients then want to take another dose to relieve the medication-induced discomfort. That is why this benzodiazepine is periodically noted for increasing the likelihood of addiction in susceptible individuals—it can leave an unfulfilled yearning for relief. Alprazolam is usually dosed two to four times a day as needed because of its abrupt end of dose offset of action. If a patient is requiring alprazolam four times a day, it may make sense for a prescriber to suggest a longer acting medication with a smoother offset of activity to avoid the repetitive roller-coaster pattern of intermittent high anxiety and relief. In fact, because of its quick onset of action, similar to diazepam, alprazolam has a street value and can be abused, sold or bought "on the street." On the other hand, alprazolam can be taken sublingually, so it may benefit those who cannot easily swallow pills.

LORAZEPAM (ATIVAN)

The length of time it takes for lorazepam to reach its therapeutic relief effect (onset), and the length time that lorazepam continues to have its desired effect (length of action), is considered middle of the road compared to other medications discussed in this chapter. The longer onset of action makes lorazepam less favorable than alprazolam for those who have panic attacks and who hope for fast relief. But its smoother winding down of action means that there is usually no rebound anxiety effect. Lorazepam is therefore likely to continue working for prolonged procedures such as MRI scans. Lorazepam also has additional effects that can be useful particularly in the cancer setting. It has been found to prevent and relieve chemotherapy-induced nausea, especially when given intravenously, and often in combination with ondansetron.[2] In addition, it helps patients who have difficulty eating because of low appetite. As noted previously, all benzodiazepines can decrease recall for events. Although this would not be beneficial if one's job required good command of facts, or when speaking with one's physician, it is not a negative consequence for those undergoing chemotherapy. In addition, unlike most other benzodiazepines, which are metabolized in the liver, lorazepam (like oxazepam and temazepam) is cleared partially by the liver but mostly by the kidneys. It is therefore safer for those who have compromised liver function, but it is more problematic in those with poor kidney clearance.

CLONAZEPAM (KLONOPIN)

Clonazepam is a longer acting minor tranquilizer. However, it also takes more time than alprazolam to begin to relieve anxiety. The advantage of this combination of pharmacodynamics is that it is less addictive because there is less immediate gratification reinforcement. The longer acting, smoother finish of its antianxiety effect leads to less rebound anxiety. Therefore, there is less of a relative discrepancy between relief and anxiety states and thus less need to find relief again very soon after the anxiety-provoking situation has passed. The longer acting nature of clonazepam can lead to a hangover or groggy feeling. Clonazepam works well to relieve panic attacks, even with its slower onset of action. Because it is longer acting, clonazepam helps people sleep longer at night. If sleep is hampered by anxious ruminations, clonazepam provides sedation and an antianxiety benefit. Clonazepam comes in a disintegrating wafer form so that patients who have difficulty swallowing pills should not have a problem with this medication.

DIAZEPAM (VALIUM)

Diazepam was an early benzodiazepine anxiolytic introduced in the 1960s. Like alprazolam, the effects of diazepam are experienced very quickly—it has a brief period of onset and a street value. However, it is also like clonazepam in that it is long acting. It too has multiple uses with impact on many parts of the body. In addition to helping sleep and anxiety, it has been used as an antiseizure medication, as can most benzodiazepines, as well as a muscle relaxant. It can cause amnesia, so it is not a recommended treatment for performance anxiety. For example, if a medication causes an actor to forget their lines, or clouds discriminatory thinking for students taking examinations, it will not lead to successful performance by decreasing anxiety. A β-blocker such as propranolol would be a better choice.

Other Benzodiazepines for Anxiety

There are other medications in the benzodiazepine family that are not used often in the oncology setting. We discuss a few of them here in case you run across them. Oxazepam is a short-acting benzodiazepine. Like lorazepam, it is initially metabolized in the liver and then excreted through the kidneys. Oxazepam is helpful in those with liver dysfunction such as alcoholics who are going through withdrawal. Midrange to longer acting benzodiazepines are usually preferred for alcohol withdrawal so that the medication has a chance to slowly taper itself between doses. Most of the longer acting benzodiazepines (i.e., diazepam, clonazepam, and chlordiazepoxide) are primarily metabolized in the liver. Librium has been a staple benzodiazepine used for alcohol withdrawal because of its sedating properties and its ability to last for longer periods of time. That it can be given intravenously like diazepam and lorazepam makes it a useful treatment in alcohol withdrawal for people who cannot take oral medications. Clorazepate (Tranxene) is a midrange-acting benzodiazepine with moderate sedating components. The last benzodiazepine we mention in this section is discussed in more detail in Chapter 4. Temazepam (Restoril) is an excellent sleep medication that is primarily excreted through the kidneys like lorazepam and oxazepam. It therefore differs from most of the other sleep medications, which are primarily metabolized in the liver. Its length of action closely mirrors the 6–8 hours patients want for a good night's sleep. Again, the caveats about dependence and tolerance must be reiterated because using these medications on a regular basis will potentially lead to problems in the future.

CASE: JIM

Now that we have learned about the different aspects of benzodiazepines from short to longer onset and offset of action and from shorter acting to longer acting, can we look back and say that lorazepam was a good choice for Jim? Although alprazolam might have had a faster onset, the abrupt cessation of its antianxiety effect might have caused problems in the middle of the night as its sedating and calming effects wore off. Also, although it might have antinausea effects, there is more clinical reliability with lorazepam. Lorazepam also seems to have been a better choice than clonazepam. Clonazepam does not usually have a fast onset of action, but it generally has a longer lasting effect. Although we could not have known this before Jim's trial with the medication, it seems like clonazepam could have had an effect for too many hours and caused similar or worse morning hangover effects for Jim than lorazepam. Anecdotally, many clinicians find that alprazolam, diazepam, and clonazepam treat panic symptoms better than lorazepam. However, given the questions initially of akathisia and nausea versus panic, the oncologist made an excellent educated choice.

Another Feature to Consider

Jim has a history of using marijuana. Is there a concern for Jim's providers about substance abuse when considering a benzodiazepine prescription? Would a non-benzodiazepine that is less habit-forming be a better alternative?

In Jim's case, a benzodiazepine was appropriate for the immediate relief of his akathisia and nausea, as well as giving fast relief of insomnia. It was also indicated given that the cause of Jim's anxiety was still within the window for benzodiazepine withdrawal. A non-benzodiazepine would not have helped. Once the medical causes of shortness of breath were ruled out, it was safe for Jim to take a benzodiazepine.

If a prescriber is concerned about substance abuse or addiction, the non-prescribing clinician may be asked to help monitor and reinforce Jim's appropriate use of the medication as well as reinforce the short-term nature of the benzodiazepine treatment. After review by all of Jim's clinicians on the appropriate use of benzos and the distinctions between dependence, tolerance, and addiction, which is often portrayed as dangerous in the media, the benzodiazepine treatment can be monitored appropriately and the drug can be used safely.

With careful oversight and monitoring by all providers, benzodiazepines have an important role in improving the quality of life of cancer patients. The non-prescriber facilitates enhanced care by observing for physical and cognitive deficits so that prescribers have additional feedback to increase confidence that the medications will not be abused or misused.

A summary of the commonly prescribed benzodiazepines used to treat anxiety in people with cancer is provided in Table 2.2 and Box 2.13, which includes useful sky view data for non-prescribers and prescribers.

THE NON-BENZODIAZEPINES FOR ANXIETY

Non-benzodiazepines such as the antidepressants, antipsychotics, buspirone, antihistamines, and the antiseizure medications such as gabapentin and pregabalin can also be used to treat or prevent chronic anxiety, as well as alleviate bothersome quality-of-life concerns such as insomnia, nausea, and pain. As with all medications, the risk:benefit ratio of taking a medication must be considered and described to patients. Some of your patients will have had long-term anxiety prior to the additional distress brought on by the uncertainties of cancer. Some might describe themselves as worriers even before the diagnosis of cancer. Some degree of worry or anxiety in the cancer setting may help promote better lifestyle changes, such as improved diet, decreased tobacco and other harmful substance intake, and greater engagement in exercise.

Table 2.2 Summary of Benzos for Anxiety in People with Cancer—Sky View

First-line medications for acute worry, phobic situations, and panic attacks. Commonly used to treat sleep problems and anxiety related to imaging scans—*scanxiety*.

Can cause drowsiness, unsteadiness, forgetfulness, and lead to falls.

If taking for more than 1 month, physical dependence can develop. *THIS IS NOT ADDICTION. DO NOT STOP ABRUPTLY!*

Taper as directed to avoid life-threatening withdrawal symptoms (e.g., seizures).

Physiological *tolerance* (needing higher doses to achieve the same relief) may develop after a few months. *THIS IS NOT ADDICTION!* But it can look like it.

Psychological addiction, or use despite harm, is rare in people who do not have addiction histories or behaviors. Use should be closely monitored in people with histories of addiction to other substances.

Alprazolam (Xanax)	Intermediate acting; best used *as needed* or for short periods of time at judicious doses. It can have an abrupt end of action experience, leading to *rebound anxiety* at the end of the therapeutic dose. Relieves intermittent panic symptoms quickly. The quick, noticeable onset of action can exacerbate *addictive behaviors.* A long-acting version of alprazolam is available.
Lorazepam (Ativan)	Moderately long acting; also used to prevent chemotherapy-induced nausea. Good for MRI anxiety. Good for those with liver dysfunction.
Diazepam (Valium)	Long acting, with quick, noticeable onset of action. This can provoke *addictive behaviors.*
Clonazepam (Klonopin)	Long acting—avoids rebound anxiety, but slower onset of action than alprazolam and diazepam. Good for panic attacks, free-floating anxiety, and inducing and maintaining sleep. Disintegrating wafer available; no swallowing needed.

Box 2.13 CONSIDERATIONS IN THE USE OF
BENZODIAZEPINES—ANOTHER VIEW

Delirium, Cognitive Impairment
Avoid benzodiazepines unless an antipsychotic medication
is already on board.

Elderly
Benzodiazepines are stored in fat cells, which are increased in
the elderly—benzodiazepines continue to clear/leach from
the system for longer periods of time and continue the active
properties until fully cleared.

Substance Abuse or Dependence
Practitioners need to take this history into account, but if
benzodiazepines are called for, use with caution, behavioral
monitoring, and education.

Central Nervous System Depression
Use caution when benzodiazepines will be given with other central nervous system depressant medications or substances (e.g.,
opioids and alcohol), potentially leading to sedation, confusion
and falls.

Respiratory Compromise
Low doses of benzodiazepines may be considered safe when
used with mild respiratory impairment, but practitioners
need to be aware of additive effects of other medications and

conditions as well as how slowly a patient might metabolize the benzodiazepine.

Caution: Intravenously administered benzodiazepines will often have more "bang for the buck" and quicker onset.

Impaired Drug Absorption and Metabolism
This can occur with all medications. Toxicity needs to be considered with altered medication absorption and metabolism.

Altered Sleep Stages
Although benzodiazepines can help induce and maintain sleep, dream states can be prolonged and intensified.

Worry may also help motivate a patient to do research and make clearer decisions about treatment choices, as well as more closely adhere to treatment regimens. Although there are many patients who take benzodiazepines on a long-term basis to treat generalized anxiety, benzos have the potential for failure over time that leads to frustration, especially if shorter acting benzos or those with abrupt offset of activity are used. Tolerance does not always occur. Some people can take the same dose of a benzodiazepine daily for years and still get the same effect. But for others, these medications suppress the anxiety for the crisis moment and for some time afterwards, but perhaps not long term. So why do these people want to keep taking benzodiazepines? It is not because they have developed a substance use disorder. Worriers are often successful, productive people. Their desire and concern for better outcomes can help them think through projects in advance and prepare for, or prevent, potential snags that could get in the way of success. On the one hand, their worry or anxiety helps achieve a better result. On the other hand, their distress does not feel good or comfortable. They may not have an easy facility to distinguish potential problems from likely problems. If concern or anxiety was not disconcerting, most would not act on it. Remember that anxiety is a signal of distress, although sometimes it may remain high even when the threat is minimal, like a faulty burglar alarm that goes off even errantly when there is no theft in progress. It can be quite exhausting to have chronic angst and worry. It is a catch-22. Benzodiazepines reduce the distress but, as discussed previously, they are limited in their ability to reduce the distress consistently over months and years. A non-benzodiazepine, such as an SSRI or SNRI antidepressant as described in Chapter 1, can have a role here.

Similarly, benzodiazepines used on an as-needed basis may relieve a panic attack but may do little to keep the next one from emerging, especially when panic attacks arise at unpredictable times. Alternatively, a medication that stays in someone's system that has antianxiety effects, such as a non-benzodiazepine, can be helpful. But that means taking the medication every day so it can build up to a therapeutic level and remain at that level to prevent generalized anxiety symptoms and panic attacks. For the most part, people will not build up tolerance to the non-benzodiazepines, so these can be taken for years and keep working.

Prescribers may also consider using non-benzodiazepines before a benzodiazepine for patients who have respiratory compromise from their cancer, from another medical issue, or from their cancer treatment, and as previously discussed, prescribers may be hesitant to suggest a benzodiazepine to someone with a history of a substance use disorder. This is an important consideration for all controlled substances and must be weighed against prognosis and severity of the patient's cancer, anxiety symptoms, as well as available alternatives.

Buspirone (Buspar) for Anxiety

Buspirone is a non-benzodiazepine anxiolytic that acts on serotonin receptors essentially increasing the levels of serotonin in the brain, much like the antidepressants. It can also enhance the dopamine neurotransmitter. Buspirone is best tolerated if titrated over a few weeks to reach a therapeutic dose. When it was first released, some prescribers were not convinced of its efficacy, perhaps because suggested dosages were too low. As is true for the antidepressants, buspirone needs to be taken daily. Like the antidepressants, it can take weeks for buspirone to take effect, making it a poor medication to treat a panic attack. Like the SSRIs and SNRIs, buspirone can be useful for generalized anxiety, with little concern for dependence, tolerance, and addiction. It can also cause gastric disturbance, so it may not be particularly helpful in someone who is struggling with nausea.

Mirtazapine (Remeron), Trazodone (Desyrel), and Other Antidepressants

Prescribers can consider using sedating antidepressants to help bring on sleep (mirtazapine or trazodone) or prevent anxiety and panic symptoms in the future. Antidepressants such as SSRIs, SNRIs, and mirtazapine need to be taken daily for at least a few weeks to treat for generalized anxiety and to prevent panic attacks from occurring, just as they do for depression. However, spontaneously taking an extra non-benzodiazepine dose will not cut short a panic attack.

ANTIPSYCHOTICS FOR ANXIETY

Olanzapine (Zyprexa) and Quetiapine (Seroquel)

When prescribers want a medication to have a relatively fast onset of action but do not want to use a benzodiazepine, they will consider an atypical antipsychotic/mood stabilizer such as olanzapine or quetiapine. For instance, when patients need help falling asleep or reducing nighttime anxiety, yet there is concern about potential confusion that can be caused by antihistamines or benzodiazepines, a sedating medication that has antianxiety properties, such as olanzapine or quetiapine can be helpful. These medications may also provide twofers by relieving chemotherapy-induced nausea and anxiety and/or insomnia due to steroid treatment.

ANTIHISTAMINES FOR ANXIETY

Antihistamines are often over-the-counter medications used to treat allergic reactions. A common side effect, especially of the older antihistamines such as diphenhydramine (Benadryl) and hydroxyzine (Atarax and Vistaril), is drowsiness. This drowsiness may induce sleep, which is why these substances are often found in sleep medications. But some people also find they get an anxiolytic response without significant drowsiness. Side effects of antihistamines include drowsiness, headache, dry mouth, skin rash, dizziness, urinary retention, constipation, and pounding heartbeat, all of which may be worse in frail or older people.

ANTISEIZURE MEDICATIONS

Gabapentin (Neurontin) and Pregabalin (Lyrica)

Two medications in the antiseizure category, gabapentin and pregabalin, have been found to be helpful to reduce anxiety in some patients. Patients with cancer who also have neuropathic pain from chemotherapy, hot flashes from hormonal treatment for prostate cancer, or insomnia may benefit from these medications, which can multitask to improve quality of life in several areas. As with many medications, the list of adverse reactions is long. However, the primary complaints from patients are somnolence, dizziness, and fatigue. As noted for other medications, starting at a lower than usual dose and slowly increasing to therapeutic levels may allow patients the time to get used to the medication and bypass the uncomfortable side effects. Evening dosing of the medication often helps improve sleep and avoid daytime sleepiness.

PROPRANOLOL FOR ANXIETY

Propranolol is a β-blocker that was used to treat hypertension decades ago. Taken long term, it was found to cause fatigue and depression, so it is not often used as an antihypertensive anymore. However, it has been found to relieve performance anxiety and panic attacks, perhaps by interfering with the tachycardic response of palpitations that can have a negative feedback effect to increase anxiety and panic. And unlike benzos, it does not cause amnesia that might impair performance, for example, on an examination or on a stage. It has also been found to help some suffering with post-traumatic stress disorder

Once the threat of benzodiazepine withdrawal passed and Jim was safely tapering off the lorazepam, the prescriber may think about suggesting a non-benzodiazepine antidepressant to prevent future panic attacks. Given the possibility that Jim was self-medicating generalized anxiety with marijuana, buspirone or an antidepressant might be excellent long-term options to help him be less anxious. The antidepressant mirtazapine might be helpful if Jim still needs a sedating medication to help him sleep; it can also be useful for ongoing anxiety control.

The antipsychotic/mood stabilizer olanzapine might also be a useful choice if Jim still has a constellation of symptoms that includes insomnia, anxiety, and nausea.

The antiseizure medications pregabalin or gabapentin may be helpful if in addition to insomnia and generalized anxiety, Jim has a neuropathic pain syndrome secondary to his chemotherapy.

Table 2.3 describes the pearls and potholes of non-benzodiazepine anxiolytics.

Table 2.3 Non-Benzodiazepine Anxiolytics

Medication	Indication	Abuse Potential
Buspirone (Buspar)	Generalized anxiety	No abuse potential
	Onset of action/ prescribing suggestions similar to those for antidepressants	
	Does not help depression, panic, or those accustomed to benzodiazepines	
	Needs to be taken daily	

Table 2.3 Continued

Medication	Indication	Abuse Potential
Antidepressants	Need to be taken daily. Beneficial effects take 2–5 weeks or longer at any one dose. *Common side effects*: anxiety, restlessness, drowsiness, and gastric upset. Antidepressants should be tapered under physician supervision to avoid discontinuation syndrome. As with use for depression, treatment lasts 9–12 months. Suicidal ideation is rare but should be mentioned to patient and monitored. May help with hot flashes for menopause or for those on hormonal treatment.	
SSRIs and SNRIs	Generalized anxiety, panic	No abuse potential
Citalopram (Celexa)		
Escitalopram (Lexapro)		

(Contniued)

Table 2.3 Continued

Medication	Indication	Abuse Potential
Fluoxetine (Prozac)		
Paroxetine (Paxil)		
Sertraline (Zoloft)		
Vortioxetine (Trintellix)		
Venlafaxine (Effexor)		
Desvenlafaxine (Pristiq)		
Mirtazapine (Remeron)	Insomnia, low appetite, no gastric upset	
Duloxetine (Cymbalta)		
Atypical Antipsychotics/ Mood Stabilizers		Can cause sedation and unsteadiness. Can cause sugar control problems, cardiac arrhythmias, and weight problems. No dependence, addiction, or need to taper.
Olanzapine (Zyprexa)	Generalized anxiety, insomnia, nausea, low appetite	No abuse potential

ANXIOLYTICS

Table 2.3 Continued

Medication	Indication	Abuse Potential
Quetiapine (Seroquel)	Generalized anxiety, insomnia	Low abuse potential (case reports)
Loxapine (Loxitane)		No abuse potential
Antihistamines		Low abuse potential
Hydroxyzine (Vistaril)	Insomnia, generalized anxiety	
Diphenhydramine (Benadryl)		
Antiseizure Medications		Low abuse potential
Pregabalin (Lyrica)	Generalized anxiety, neuropathic pain	Unclear abuse potential—higher than first thought
Gabapentin (Neurontin)	Generalized anxiety, neuropathic pain, hot flashes	Unclear abuse potential—higher than first thought
Propranolol	Performance anxiety and panic	Low abuse potential; can lower blood pressure; can cause dizziness

SNRIs, serotonin norepinephrine reuptake inhibitors; SSRIs, selective serotonin reuptake inhibitors.

INTRODUCING: JENNA

You have been doing psychotherapy with Jenna, a 56-year-old woman who completed primary treatment for breast cancer approximately 1 year ago. She is taking tamoxifen now. Jenna says she has been feeling high anxiety in anticipation of upcoming scans. Her mother, who was treated for colon cancer many years ago, was only in remission for 3 years before the cancer recurred in multiple places. Jenna denies any panic symptoms. She has tried the relaxation exercises you taught her but cannot shut the worry thoughts off, especially at night. What information would you include in your discussion with the oncology team?

A discussion with the primary treatment team about Jenna's anxiety can help the team consider whether a benzodiazepine briefly prior to getting her scans and while waiting to receive the results is a good idea or whether a non-benzodiazepine is a better choice over a longer period. Usually when patients go on a non-benzodiazepine for an anxiety or depressive disorder, they commit to treatment for at least 9 months to 1 year. Interestingly, we have observed clinically that patients with long histories of general anxiety or worry want to stay on an antidepressant beyond 1 year when prescribed for anxiety. They notice for the first time what it is like *not* to have the ongoing din of worry about what will happen, what should happen, what they fear will or will not happen, what they or others need to do or should do, or what they or others should not do. It is not that they do not care. They just worry less. Although this type of apprehension can be very helpful prior to cancer while studying in school, producing in the workplace, or completing important projects, it is less helpful when waiting for medical tests that cannot be studied for or dealing with results that often are out of a patient's control.

INTRODUCING: PETE

Pete is a 60-year-old man who has been receiving chemotherapy for recently diagnosed pancreatic cancer. He started having panic attacks a few weeks before the diagnosis. The attacks have continued every few days. Each attack lasts 10–30 minutes and consists of heart palpitations, sweating, and shortness of breath. He also experiences a foreboding sense of dread. He has been having trouble eating, complaining of mild nausea and a sense of abdominal fullness. He even visited an emergency room because he thought he was having a heart attack, but he was cleared medically. He tells the oncology team that he was confident that the chemotherapy would work, just as chemotherapy helped his mother live 5 years after a diagnosis of metastatic lung cancer even though she had an initial prognosis of less than 2 years to live. However, he is considering stopping the treatment because of the anxiety and panic: "I cannot take this anymore."

What can you discuss with the primary treating team?

Pete is experiencing panic symptoms. It has been reported that both depressive and anxiety symptoms can be related to pancreatic cancer. These symptoms can even be prodromal—that is, they manifest even before the cancer is diagnosed—or can occur afterwards. The biological mechanism of this phenomenon is still not clear, although it may be related to the cytokine protein part of the immune system. This has been seen in patients who do not have any previous history of anxiety or depressive disorders. Therapists have experienced these patients as having intractable symptoms that are not improved with various psychotherapeutic techniques. It would be beneficial for the non-prescriber to speak with the oncology team to let them know about the recalcitrance of the panic symptoms and include a description of the pattern, if any, of the symptoms, noting their quality, frequency, situational descriptions, and severity. The therapist would ask whether the symptoms might be related to any of the chemotherapy agents or other medications or supplements that the patient is taking. The therapist would want to know that the panic symptoms are not medically related, and not just assume that they are psychological. For example, abnormal thyroid functions, electrolytes, or cardiac abnormalities can cause anxiety or panic-like symptoms. The therapist would also want to know if an anxiety medication could be helpful. The oncology team may be pleased to know that the patient will be receiving ongoing therapy to deal with curtailing panic attacks and supporting compliance with all medications

INTRODUCING: MARIE

Marie is a 64-year-old woman who has been on a ventilator for complications of postoperative pneumonia after surgery for head and neck cancer. The intensive care unit (ICU) team is trying to wean her off the ventilator. She is able to write on a chalkboard, "No, no, don't take out the tube. I will die. I won't be able to breathe." She acknowledges being anxious and her fear of not being able to breathe and then dying. Although her breathing has improved, the team does not want to compromise her respiratory status with any medications that can lower respiratory drive. As the social worker on the unit, you are asked to teach the patient relaxation exercises. You show Marie how to do visualization exercises, but they do not help enough. Are there additional recommendations to discuss with the team?

Marie is experiencing anxiety about not being able to breathe without ventilator support. Every time the team has tried to wean her, she feels a change in her respiratory drive that leads to heightened worry, despite reassurances from the ICU team that she will be fine. The team members note their concern about using benzodiazepines for Marie due to potentially compromising her breathing, but they are not sure what to do. Her family has said that

PSYCHOPHARMACOLOGY IN CANCER CARE

because of a bad experience with a psychiatrist involving a family member many years ago, Marie does not want to see a psychiatrist.

The social worker talks with the primary team and sees the degree of anxiety Marie has when discussing weaning off of the ventilator. Marie has difficulty feeling her body, let alone trying to do passive muscle relaxation. They try visualizing pleasant memories of places Marie visited with her family, but she feels unable to keep focused on other parts of her body as her attention drifts quickly back to her breath, and she feels nauseated. The social worker and team recognize Marie's anxiety and nausea. The team proposes olanzapine in the wafer formulation to help relieve her symptoms but not compromise her breathing.

SUMMARY

Prescribers and non-prescribers should not be fearful of using benzodiazepines or other antianxiety medications to help cancer patients cope with anxiety. When considering how to improve quality of life, there is the right time for the right medication in the right patient. Frailty, respiratory status, a history of and current substance use, the nature of a patient's anxiety, and response to psychotherapeutic interventions will all be taken into consideration in deciding when to consider a medication to treat anxiety and which one.

NOTES

1. See https://adaa.org/about-adaa/press-room/facts-statistics.
2. Buzdar AU, Esparza L, Natale R, et al. Lorazepam-enhancement of the antiemetic efficacy of dexamethasone and promethazine: A placebo-controlled study. *Am J Clin Oncol.* 1994;17(5):417–421.

Chapter 3

Antipsychotics

Managing Delirium, Anxiety, and Nausea

INTRODUCTION

The uses for antipsychotics may be much different in a cancer setting than in a non-cancer setting. In a cancer population, these medications are primarily used to help manage the symptoms and side effects of cancer or cancer treatment, such as delirium, confusion, agitation, anxiety, insomnia, or nausea. When an antipsychotic is started in the cancer setting, the prescriber may clarify with the patient and family that the medication in this situation is *not* for schizophrenia or bipolar disorder as the package insert or online information lists for preponderant uses.

The most common reason to use an antipsychotic for patients with cancer is to manage delirium. Because delirium is one of the principal reasons for a psycho-oncology consult in the inpatient setting, this chapter focuses mainly on delirium and how best to manage it. It also discusses the role of antipsychotics in helping manage anxiety, insomnia, manic episodes and nausea.

Delirium is a medical emergency. Because delirium is a manifestation of an underlying medical problem, the situation is likely to get worse if not attended to. Therefore, it is important for non-prescribing clinicians to be able to identify delirium and cognitive changes that might be addressed medically and perhaps managed by an antipsychotic medication in their patients with cancer. Likewise, it is also important to recognize side effects of antipsychotics that may impair a patient's functioning. Again, you may be the first responder or the most frequent monitor of a patient's quality of life and reactions to various medications.

The primary way to deal with a delirious patient is to understand and treat the causes of the delirium. That means first and foremost to understand that a patient who may look agitated, anxious, depressed, lethargic, or confused may have an underlying medical cause of those symptoms that, if ameliorated, can relieve the other symptoms. However, even experienced clinicians do not always recognize that a delirium is the proper diagnosis, and therefore the steps to resolving it get delayed. Sometimes the delirium can be exacerbated or prolonged by incorrect or delayed identification and, therefore, incorrect management (e.g., treating an anxious symptom of delirium with a benzodiazepine that worsens a patient's confusion).

TOPICS TO ADDRESS WITH PATIENTS, SO THEY CAN ASK THEIR PRESCRIBERS

Non-prescribers may be the first observers of the early phases of a delirium or a cognitive disorder related to a patient's cancer or cancer treatment. You can query the patient to further explore your observations and alert the oncology team about your concerns. Delirium is common in cancer patients, especially in the inpatient setting, although it is often not recognized until its symptoms are florid, and perhaps dangerous, to the health of the patient or the safety of others. As with all illnesses, the earlier a problem is recognized, the better the odds of resolution. The sooner a delirium is diagnosed, the faster the underlying medical problem can be addressed and the earlier the symptoms can be alleviated.

Non-prescribers can reinforce to patients and family members that an antipsychotic used for delirium is likely not being prescribed as in the general psychiatric population, assuming the patients does not have an underlying major psychiatric disorder such as schizophrenia or bipolar disorder. This is especially important if the patient is hesitant to take a medication because they heard it was for psychiatric patients. Clarifying that treatment with an antipsychotic does not mean a person has suddenly developed a major psychiatric disorder or, as discussed later, even psychosis, can be reassuring.

Patients discharged from the inpatient oncology ward after treatment for delirium may be seen as outpatients by non-prescribers, even before these patients see their primary oncologists. These patients may also be seen by non-prescribers more often than by the oncology team. Thus, non-prescribers are in an excellent position to note possible antipsychotic side effects, such as daytime sedation or ambulation difficulties, as well as the effectiveness of the medication and alert the oncology team.

As mentioned previously, patients do not have to be psychotic to receive an antipsychotic. They may be on antipsychotic-like medications for non-psychiatric purposes such as to relieve nausea (i.e., metoclopramide and prochlorperazine) or on atypical antipsychotics such as olanzapine or quetiapine for nausea, insomnia, anxiety, or cognitive clouding. Non-prescribers do their patients a service by understanding the scope and impact of treatment with these medications. Given the number of prescribers seen by patients during hospital stays and in outpatient care, and the potential for suboptimal communication when transitioning to the outpatient setting, the non-prescriber may have the most consistent relationship of all a patient's formal caregivers.

AVOIDING THE POTHOLES OF DIAGNOSING AGITATION, CONFUSION, AND LETHARGY IN CANCER PATIENTS

From Delirium and Cognitive Disorders to Anxiety, Insomnia, Nausea, and Poor Appetite—Sometimes a Diagnosis Is Not Easy to Make

Non-prescribers do not commonly come across confused cancer patients in their outpatient practices. More often, confusion is noted in the inpatient setting when patients are sicker medically. Oncology patients can become confused for many reasons, such as cancer's effect on the brain via metastatic lesions or a paraneoplastic syndrome, a rare clinical condition in cancer characterized by a nonmetastatic, but distant, reaction to the tumor or antibodies produced by the tumor, may also be at risk for confusion disorders and require antipsychotic medication to resolve uncomfortable or frightening symptoms. These abnormal responses can influence parts of the brain, spinal cord, neuromuscular structures, as well as the endocrine, dermatologic, blood, or rheumatologic systems. Other causes for confusion include side effects of medications, physiological anomalies, and medical comorbidities. Thus, non-prescribing clinicians such as psychotherapists, and occupational and physical therapists, will see people with cancer in both the inpatient and the outpatient setting who are susceptible to confusion and delirium. As they visit patients in the hospital, clinicians may find that patients are cognitively impaired, sedated, or not able to attend to instructions or conversations clearly. Similarly, in the outpatient setting, patients may have had recent delirious experiences prior to hospital discharge, and non-prescribers may hear about the fear of losing cognitive control or even of having to re-enter the hospital. Prescribers who are not psycho-oncologists may come across people at risk for delirium, or patients who have experienced delirium, and may be able to investigate potential causes that can be remediated, such as aberrant labs or side effects of a medication.

Delirium is an acute neuropsychiatric disturbance that can be caused by numerous medical etiologies. Delirium is characterized by poor attention, cognitive difficulties such as disorientation, thought disorder, or perceptual problems such as hallucinations or paranoid ideation. It can be marked by restlessness and agitation or combativeness (hyperactive) or lethargy (hypoactive) or a mixed state of both.

RISK FACTORS FOR SYNDROMES OF DELIRIUM OR CONFUSION IN CANCER PATIENTS

People who are more susceptible to having delirium include the elderly, the medically frail, and patients who are dehydrated, with or without substantial electrolyte abnormalities. Patients with compromised brain function and those with significant cardiovascular, pulmonary, liver, or renal dysfunction are also more prone to episodes of confusion. Side effects to various medications and immunosuppression can also increase risk for delirium or confusion. Medical comorbidities, medications, and cancer treatments that can increase the risk of confusion in cancer patients is listed in Boxes 3.1–3.3.

Box 3.1 COMORBIDITIES THAT CAN INCREASE THE RISK OF CONFUSION IN CANCER PATIENTS

- Infections/sepsis
- Strokes
- Hypoxia/anemia
- Brain tumors (primary or metastatic)
- Hepatic dysfunction
- Kidney dysfunction
- Emboli
- Seizures
- Leptomeningeal disease
- Paraneoplastic syndromes
- Electrolyte abnormalities/dehydration
- Hypercalcemia
- Endocrine abnormalities (e.g., hyper-/hypothyroid)
- Nutritional/vitamin abnormalities
  - B_{12} deficiency
  - Thiamine deficiency

Box 3.2 POTENTIAL MEDICATION/SUBSTANCE
CAUSES OF CONFUSION

- Postoperative effects of anesthesia
- Substance intoxication or withdrawal
- Sleep medications
- Benzodiazepines
- Pain medications (opioids)
- Steroids (even those given as adjuvant to chemotherapy)
- Medications with anticholinergic effects
  - Ifosfamide (Ifex): Chemotherapy used to treat testicular cancer, sarcomas, and lymphomas
  - Trimetrexate (Neutrexin): An anti-infective agent used to treat pneumonia in immunocompromised patients
- Serotonin syndrome: Caused by various medications that increase serotonin levels
- Neuroleptic malignant syndrome: Usually caused by antipsychotic medications that decrease central dopamine
- Acyclovir and amphotericin B: Antiviral medications
- Drug interactions
- P450 interactions/abnormal albumin levels
- Syndrome of inappropriate antidiuretic hormone secretion (SIADH): A situation in which the body makes too much ADH, which is produced in the hypothalamus. This leads to abnormal kidney control of fluid volume. SIADH can be caused by medications, infections, strokes, and lung disease, including pneumonia, as well as cancers of the lung, pancreas, and small intestine.
- Abnormal glucose

Box 3.3 CANCER TREATMENTS THAT CAN CAUSE CONFUSION

- Chemotherapy agents
  - Methotrexate, 5-flurouracil, bleomycin, cisplatin, asparaginase, procarbazine, ifosfamide, capecitabine, carboplatin, cytarabine, trimetrexate
- Radiation therapy side effects

IDENTIFYING A SYNDROME OF DELIRIUM IN CANCER PATIENTS

Unfortunately, there is no good algorithm for diagnosing delirium, but we present one in Box 3.4. Asking the question, "What's wrong with this picture?" and awareness of the possibility of delirium are the best ways to be prepared to recognize it if it is present. Remember that identifying delirium will not fix the problem. Fixing whatever is causing the delirium will fix the delirium. Sometimes the symptoms of delirium may be the only indication that some underlying medical issue is awry, and practitioners will have to wait to see whether delirium develops and to identify what medical abnormality needs to be corrected.

Box 3.4 ALGORITHM FOR THINKING THAT A DELIRIUM MAY
BE PRESENT

When anxiety or depressed mood seem to be
unexplained, in terms of intensity or temporal
appearance, and develop over hours to days
OR
When someone develops disorientation over hours to days
OR
When someone becomes agitated or restless, out of
proportion to the situation over hours to days
OR
When someone becomes lethargic or is intermittently
alert and hyperaroused over hours to days
OR
When someone is uncharacteristically acutely combative
over hours to days
OR
When someone starts hallucinating (usually visual) over
hours to days
OR
When someone becomes paranoid over hours to days
OR
When someone's alertness or mental status fluctuates
among some or all of the above entities
Think about delirium!

CAN DELIRIUM BE PREVENTED?

Studies have examined whether the prophylactic use of medication can decrease the incidence of delirium. These medications have included antipsychotics, cholinesterase inhibitors, dexmedetomidine, melatonin, and ramelteon. Thus far, there is mixed evidence of efficacy for these methods of preventing delirium or improving clinical outcomes. Trials have also been undertaken to determine if terminal delirium in dying patients can be prevented, but, again, results have been inconsistent. It is beyond the scope of this psychopharmacologic primer to discuss this topic in further detail. However, it is useful to keep this in mind when caring for a patient who is frail or who has experienced delirium previously and who requires a surgical procedure or hospitalization that may carry a high risk of delirium. If you know a patient has a history of previous delirium, share it with the oncologist and other prescribers. It is important for all caregivers to consider decreasing the number of avoidable medications patients are prescribed, as the potential for drug–drug interactions that can cause delirium is exacerbated.

CHALLENGES OF DIAGNOSING DELIRIUM IN PEOPLE WITH CANCER—LOOK-ALIKES

Delirium may be considered a diagnostic masquerader. Although delirium is caused acutely by a medical problem, its presentation can mimic dementia (cognitive deficits and/or disorientation with or without perceptual disturbances), anxiety (acute excessive worry or restlessness), depression (emotional lability, such as excessive or out-of-proportion crying, sadness, or psychomotor retardation), or mania

Table 3.1 Distinguishing Delirium from Dementia

	Delirium	*Dementia*
Onset and duration	Usually acute, hours to days	Ongoing, progressing slowly over months to years
Sensorium (alertness)	Waxing and waning; variations in alertness	Clear
Attention	May be disrupted or fragmented	Clear
Thoughts	Disorganized, incoherent	Impoverished in later stages
Perceptions	Hallucinations (visual > auditory)	May be present
Psychomotor behavior	Hyper- or hypoactive (agitated or sluggish or lethargic)	Usually unchanged; it is not uncommon for delirium to be superimposed on dementia

(disinhibition, irritability, agitation, or combativeness). A hallmark of delirium is impaired attention and a waxing and waning of a patient's sensorium, or degree of alertness, that has a relatively acute onset. Table 3.1 provides hints to distinguish delirium from dementia.

It is not unusual for the non-prescribing provider to be asked to evaluate a cancer patient for depression, when in fact the underlying problem is a (hypoactive) delirium. Distinguishing depression from a delirium, as illustrated in Table 3.2, is facilitated by assessing the rapidity of onset of symptoms, the presence of a disturbance of sensorium (alertness) and attention, new or worsening cognitive

Table 3.2 Distinguishing Delirium from Depression

	Delirium (Hypoactive)	Depression
Onset	Abrupt	Slow, most of the day, most days of the week for more than 2 weeks
Sensorium/ attention	Waxing and waning; variations in alertness	Clear
Cognition/ thoughts	Disorganized, incoherent	Mood congruent delusions with hopelessness, guilt, and worthlessness themes
Perceptual changes	Visual hallucinations	Auditory hallucinations, often derogatory, self-deprecating
Mood	May appear sad, labile, disinhibited	Depressed mood with anhedonia, hopelessness, worthlessness, and possible suicidal ideation
Suicidality	Impulsive, sometimes associated with delusions	May predate the current presentation—important to ask about it
Past psychiatric history	Possible history of delirium	Possible history of depression
Family psychiatric history	Unknown	Possible history of depression, bipolar disorder, or suicidality

deficits, the presence and type of perceptual disturbances, as well as past psychiatric and family psychiatric history.

ASK, BECAUSE THEY MAY NOT TELL; TELL BEFORE THEY ASK

Myths That Keep Cancer Patients from Taking Antipsychotics

"I don't have schizophrenia."

"First I find out I have cancer. Now my doctors think I have a major mental disorder."

"My grandmother used to take Thorazine and had lots of uncontrollable movements. They called it tardive dyskinesia. I don't need any more problems!"

Antipsychotics in a cancer setting are not generally used for schizophrenia unless this was a pre-existing condition. With cancer patients, antipsychotics are generally given at lower doses and for shorter periods of time compared to the non-cancer setting; as a result, the side effect profile in cancer patients tends to be more tolerable than that in non-cancer patients. Antipsychotics will be used to control the psychosis or agitation of delirium until the underlying medical process can be corrected, if possible.

If an antipsychotic is used for a purpose other than psychosis, the patient may not realize to which class it belongs until they read the package insert. So, after you find out what medications have been suggested to the patient by the prescriber, let them know what you know about the medication, hopefully before they read the package insert.

MEDS FOR HEADS

Box 3.5 lists the most commonly used antipsychotics in the cancer setting so you can start to gain familiarity with the generic and brand names. We could add prochlorperazine (Compazine) and metoclopramide (Reglan) to this list because they are chemically similar to the antipsychotic medications and have similar side effect

---

Box 3.5 ANTIPSYCHOTICS OFTEN USED IN THE CANCER
SETTING

Generic Name of Medication	Brand Name of Medication
Haloperidol	Haldol
Olanzapine	Zyprexa
Quetiapine	Seroquel
Risperidone	Risperdal
Chlorpromazine	Thorazine
Aripiprazole	Abilify
Ziprasidone	Geodon
Asenapine	Saphrys, Sycrest
Lurasidone	Latuda

---

profiles. However, these two medications are used primarily for antinausea effects and do not treat psychosis, so they are not included.

Box 3.6 describes the multiple situations in which antipsychotics might be used in the cancer setting.

Box 3.6 USES FOR ANTIPSYCHOTICS IN THE CANCER
SETTING

- Schizophrenia or bipolar disorders that predate the cancer diagnosis
- Psychotic symptoms from any etiology
- Agitation or irritability from delirium or medications
- Mood stabilization from manic episode or medications
- Anxiety, especially if benzodiazepines are contraindicated
- Anxiety related to ventilator weaning
- Insomnia
- Nausea from multiple causes
- Poor appetite

INTRODUCING: JOE

Joe is a 56-year-old man who was recently diagnosed with colo-rectal cancer. You saw him a few months before his surgery for anxiety and coping. His mother died of colon cancer 20 years ago in her 50s, and his father died of a heart attack when Joe was aged 20 years. Joe was afraid of dying and worried that he would not be able to see his three daughters, who are in their 20s, get married and have children. He is a muscular but overweight successful car salesman who has a couple of beers a day after work with friends or co-workers. He had never seen a therapist previously, but a friend who appreciated your help coping with his own lung cancer suggested he see you, as Joe was drinking more rather than reducing his alcohol use prior to surgery. You did supportive therapy to help prepare Joe psychologically and even physically for his surgery, having him slowly reduce his alcohol use to a few beers per week.

Joe comes back to see you approximately 2 months after being discharged postoperatively to tell you the good news on his pathology report, but he does not understand why he feels so anxious. Joe tells you that his surgery was complicated by an infection that required a few days in the intensive care unit (ICU). He says he still feels a little foggy, and during the past week he was more nervous than he was before his surgery. "It doesn't make sense; I should be happy."

You do a cognitive screen on Joe because of his "foggy" feeling and compare it to the screen you did as a baseline prior to surgery. He has some attention deficits and mild recall difficulties that were not present previously. He looks more tired but has difficulty sitting still. Joe's speech is slower than in the past, and he insists he has not had any beer since his surgery. He thinks he is just tired from his recuperation and is just a bit short of breath.

You wonder if Joe is just experiencing ongoing recovery from his surgery and complicated hospital course, but you are concerned about his new cognitive problems. His degree of alertness and quick-wittedness is not what it was before surgery. While Joe is in your office, you call his surgeon, who recommends Joe come to the emergency room.

Although it is not clear to you as a non-prescriber whether Joe has a delirium or a new or recurrent underlying medical or neurological problem, it is clear that Joe looks, sounds, and is acting differently than before. Joe's cognitive screen today is worrisome, and you are grateful that you did a baseline examination on him months ago, even though he said he was "sharp as a tack" and had indeed sailed through the 5-minute examination then. You later receive feedback from Joe's oncologist that he indeed had developed another infection; he had a pulmonary embolus; he had an electrolyte imbalance, possibly because of difficulty eating after surgery; and he had signs of delirium. Nice detective work and action!

WHAT MIGHT TIP A PRESCRIBER TO SUGGEST AN ANTIPSYCHOTIC MEDICATION? AND WHY WOULD A NON-PRESCRIBER WANT TO KNOW?

Because delirium is a manifestation of an underlying medical problem, the medical situation needs to be attended to quickly, or it is likely to get worse. Delirious patients can become agitated and combative. Patients, family, and medical staff are at risk of being injured by a patient who is acutely disoriented, combative, paranoid, or hallucinating. Although the primary team will want to correct the underlying medical problem as soon as possible, antipsychotics can relieve the symptoms that could lead to violence and injury or impede the medical workup necessary to understand the underlying anomaly and fix it. Therefore, the sooner any health care professional who treats the patient can alert the primary team to the possibility of a delirium, the sooner medications such as antipsychotics can be given to calm the patient and treat some of the manifestations of delirium so that a medical workup can begin. Likewise, it is also important to recognize side effects of antipsychotics that may impair a patient's functioning. You may be the first responder or the most frequent monitor of a patient's quality of life and reactions to various medications.

When you ask patients what medications they take, it is important to ask if they are taking antipsychotics. Patients may not offer that information spontaneously, thinking in a parallel way, "Why does my therapist need to know what I am taking for nausea?" or "I am seeing my therapist to help me cope with dying. What does a medication for confusion caused by an infection in the hospital a week ago have to do with that?" or "I don't want people to know that I am taking a medication for schizophrenia." You, as a non-prescriber or as a non-psycho-oncology prescriber, will be able to use your clinical skills of surveillance to look for side effects, which, if present, can be most compromising to the patient's quality of life. If the patient questions your inquiry, you can state that monitoring and observing the patient can greatly increase the speed of identification and resolution of disability or distress, expanding the care of their oncology team. You can also explain how some physical symptoms, such as fatigue, may be related to the patient's recent hospitalization but may also be related to ongoing or fluctuating symptoms of delirium or to side effects of continuing antipsychotic treatment.

On an inpatient medical unit, if your patient does not have a history of delirium but appears cognitively clouded or disoriented, it is helpful to notify the primary oncology team members so they can more quickly identify the cause of the cognitive problem and, perhaps address it without any psychopharmacologic intervention.

Rule of Thumb

It bears repeating that the way to resolve a delirium is to fix the underlying cause of the delirium—the cause is medical, so the remedy is medical. The psychiatric aspects of delirium, such as combativeness, impulsivity, agitation, hallucinations, or paranoia, are important symptoms to address because they can interfere with the medical workup and treatment and can make the hospital environment unsafe for patients and staff. Treating the symptoms of a hypoactive delirium such as confusion or psychotic symptoms in a patient who is lethargic and has psychomotor slowing is also important because the nature of a delirium can change abruptly. Someone who appears "pleasantly confused" can become agitated and aggressive quickly, leading to patient fear and impulsivity and potential danger to the patient, family, other patients, and staff. Perceptual disturbances such as paranoid delusions or hallucinations can be frightening to the patient, family, and staff. It is wise to treat even pleasant hallucinations because they can turn into frightening ones without warning and are nevertheless the result of an underlying medical problem.

CASE: JOE

Joe is readmitted to the hospital, and within a few hours he becomes irritable and says he is "sure the cancer has come back" and that he wants to die because he cannot go through more treatment: "I have been through enough." He is being treated for a pulmonary embolus and pneumonia. A social work colleague is asked to see Joe because of Joe's suicidal statement. Your colleague's assessment reveals cognitive dysfunction as well as mood lability with irritability and anxiety. Joe is suspicious but without any fixed paranoid delusions, and has no hallucinations.

Your colleague informs you of the findings, and you are both concerned that this is a delirium. Joe is put on a 1:1 constant observation for safety as the oncology team addresses the delirium. Psychiatry is called and recommends olanzapine 2.5 mg now with a second dose at bedtime. After the psychiatrist obtains a more detailed history, she finds that during Joe's last hospitalization and ICU stay, he was confused and received haloperidol. Because his medical situation resolved quickly, the haloperidol was discontinued. Joe did not remember that his ICU stay included having a mild delirium. The psychiatrist suggests olanzapine because it can address Joe's agitation, but tells the oncology team that it may have mild anticholinergic effects, in case that might still be an issue for slowing Joe's bowel function. She also suggests haloperidol as needed if Joe becomes more agitated. A private room is recommended for Joe so his wife can stay the night and also so he does not disturb other patients. The nursing staff is asked to do frequent reorientation with Joe.

THE BENEFITS OF NON-PHARMACOLOGIC STRATEGIES FOR DELIRIUM

Although this book is about psychopharmacology, non-pharmacologic strategies for delirium may be welcome by primary oncology team prescribers and non-prescribers on inpatient medical units (Box 3.7). Non-prescribers in the hospital setting can review with the primary team and family members important approaches that will help provide a safe and supportive environment for patient, staff, and family.

Box 3.7 NON-PHARMACOLOGIC INTERVENTIONS
FOR DELIRIUM

- Reassurance to, and communication with, family, educating about delirium
- Well-lit room
- Visible clock
- Visible calendar
- Frequent reorientation
- Familiar people, objects, and photos
- Early mobilization
- Encourage hydration
- Assess for poor nutrition
- Assess for pain and hypoxia
- Sensory aids for hearing and vision

Non-prescribers can also provide reassurance to family about the medical and likely transient nature of delirium, unless the patient is near end of life. These strategies include a well-lit room; a visible clock; a visible calendar; frequent reorientation; familiar people, objects, and photos; early mobilization; and communicating with the patient and family about the goals of care and desirable outcomes (e.g., sedation vs. awake but agitated, or with hallucinations).

How Antipsychotic Medications Work, and Why It Is Important for Non-Prescribers and Patients to Know Too

Non-prescribers can support family and patients with information about symptomatic treatment with antipsychotics to control delusions, hallucinations, or agitation in the cancer setting. You can explain why some tranquilizing medications, such as benzodiazepines, may not be used for delirium (they can make confusion worse). Your explanations and support will clarify why these psychiatric medications are being used in this cancer setting.

The neurophysiology of delirium is complicated, with many brain transmitter systems implicated, including dopamine, acetylcholine, and γ-aminobutyric acid receptors, as well as excess glutamate activity. Antipsychotics block certain dopaminergic transmission in various areas of the brain. Dopamine has a role in the reward system of the brain, thus being implicated in addiction chemistry, but also in how people respond to significant stimuli. Abnormal dopamine transmission alters these processes, leading to a problematic sense of novelty and inappropriate assignment of importance that can lead to the experience of perceptual disturbances. Antipsychotics improve delusional thoughts and hallucinations by blocking the dopamine receptors in several brain regions by diminishing abnormal transmissions. Dopamine blockades that occur nonspecifically can lead to unintentional hazards (e.g., parkinsonian symptoms occur because dopamine receptors are blocked in the substantia nigra portion of the basal ganglia that controls motor movements).

The side effects of antipsychotics are varied and include restlessness, sedation, confusion, urinary and bowel dysfunction, as well as neuro-muscular dysfunction such as parkinsonism as noted above, with extra-pyramidal symptoms and gait disturbance. For this class of medication, as with so many others, if we only considered the side effects, we may never take or prescribe them. But the benefits are extremely important. Anticholinesterase inhibitors (used to manage dementia) as well as α_2 agonists (used to treat hypertension) have been used to treat delirium as well. However, they have not shown consistent benefits. To date, there is no US Food and Drug Administration-approved medication class for treatment of delirium. The American Psychiatric Association's guidelines for treating delirium recommend antipsychotics at low doses for short periods of time with close monitoring for adverse effects, espe-cially in older medically frail patients.[1]

Haloperidol was developed in the 1950s. It was used as a treatment for the psychotic symptoms of schizophrenia and bipolar disorder. In the cancer setting, it is primarily used to treat the agitation and psy-chotic symptoms of delirium. It has been thought of as the "go-to" antipsychotic for delirious medically ill patients because of its ease of administration (by mouth, intramuscularly, or intravenously).

A Cochrane database review suggested that haloperidol and selected atypical antipsychotics such as olanzapine and risperidone are effective in managing the symptoms of delirium, although there were too few randomized control trials to complete a significant meta-analysis.[2] A more recent review found no reported data to determine whether antipsychotics altered the duration of delirium, length of hospital stay, or health-related quality of life given poor quality of these studies and reporting of these symptoms.[3]

We believe one of the most significant studies on the treatment of delirium in cancer patients was done by Breitbart in 1996[4] in people with HIV and HIV-related cancers. The study found that haloperidol alone and chlorpromazine alone each improved symptoms of delirium better than lorazepam, a benzodiazepine, which often made the symptoms worse.

We previously stated that antipsychotic medications used for delirium differ in terms of dose and duration compared with their use in the general psychiatric population for psychotic or mood disorders. Non-prescribers can help patients and families understand the alarming black box warnings that exist for all antipsychotic medications cautioning about potential cerebral vascular accidents, strokes, and prolongation of cardiac conduction, especially in older adults with a history of dementia. Non-prescribers can point out that side effects occur more frequently at higher doses, which are more common with primary psychotic disorders, and less often at the lower doses used for controlling the symptoms of delirium. Unfortunately, idiosyncratic reactions can occur at any dose. Non-prescribers can clarify why electrocardiograms are checked periodically to monitor for slowed cardiac conduction. Cardiac monitoring and examining for parkinsonian symptoms can raise worries about negative outcomes. Non-prescribers can remind families about the risk:benefit ratio of any medication and that the potential consequences of a prolonged delirium are serious. They can also be reassuring from the perspective of identifying potential problems sooner rather than later, so the oncology team has appropriate information to pivot tactics if needed, rather than being caught by surprise and perhaps when it is too late.

The black box warnings also suggest caution about atypical antipsychotics' potential to cause glucose intolerance, diabetes, and ketoacidosis. These side effects are not common unless patients are taking the medications over longer periods of time. Patients who already have diabetes or who are on steroids may be at higher risk for these syndromes.

Non-prescribers can also help the primary team reduce factors that may contribute to, or exacerbate, the potential harm from delirium by notifying the treatment team whether patients are on multiple different medications from various prescribers (especially when patients have multiple prescribers in multiple, but not connected, facilities). Such medications might include opioids, sleep medications, or anticholinergic medications (over-the-counter or prescribed), as well as supplements, or if the patient has had recent substance intoxication, or may be having substance withdrawal.

UNDERSTANDING THE STRATEGIES OF THE PSYCHO-ONCOLOGY MEDICATION PRESCRIBER

How a Prescriber Thinks About Prescribing an Anti-Psychotic Medication in the Cancer Setting

THE MEDESCORT GUIDE FOR ANTIPSYCHOTICS

Table 3.3 lists the antipsychotics most likely to be used to treat delirium. It summarizes routes of administration, starting dosages, and

Table 3.3 Antipsychotics Used to Treat Symptoms of Delirium

Medication	Route of Administration	Starting Dosages	Sky View Pearls and Potholes
Haloperidol	PO; IM; IV	0.5–2 mg; 5 mg for severe	Risk of EPS; monitor QTc
Olanzapine	PO; Zydis wafer	2.5–5 mg q 12 hours prn	Atypical; monitor QTc
Quetiapine	PO	25–150 mg q 12 hours prn	Atypical; monitor QTc
Risperidone	PO; M-tab	0.25–3 mg q 12 hours prn	Uncontrolled muscle movements or weakness; EPS
Chlorpromazine	PO; IM; IV	12.5–50 mg q 4–12 hours prn	Sedating; anticholinergic; monitor QTc
Aripiprazole	PO	5–15 mg daily	Energizing
Ziprasidone	PO; IM	20–80 mg Q 12 hours prn	Monitor QTc
Asenapine	PO; sublingual	5 mg daily	Sublingual; good for those who cannot swallow
Lurasidone	PO	20 mg daily	P450 3A4 interactions; can be sedating

EPS, extrapyramidal symptoms—parkinsonism; IM, intramuscularly; IV, intravenously; M tab, orally disintegrating tablet; PO, by mouth; prn, as needed; QTc, cardiac conduction measure; Zydis, orally disintegrating tablet—still requires swallowing.

provides a sky view column to highlight pearls and potholes of these medications.

Prescribers can consider many variables when they intend to prescribe an antipsychotic medication to a patient with cancer. Information that a non-prescriber may find helpful is included in Box 3.8.

Box 3.8 QUESTIONS PRESCRIBERS CONSIDER FOR CHOOSING THE "RIGHT" ANTIPSYCHOTIC

Has the patient responded to an antipsychotic in the past?

Has the patient had a side effect to an antipsychotic medication in the past?

Can the patient take medications by mouth and swallow?

Is the patient calm enough to take a medication by mouth?

Is the patient too agitated or combative to take a medication by mouth?

Does the patient require sedation for safety?

Is the patient having difficulty sleeping at night?

Is the patient complaining of nausea?

Is the patient complaining of anxiety but cannot take a benzodiazepine?

Does the patient have significant bowel slowing or obstruction?

Does the patient have a significant cardiac history or prolonged QTc?

Is the patient already overly sedated or at risk for falls?

Did the patient have parkinsonian symptoms before starting an antipsychotic?

HOW ANTIPSYCHOTICS ARE USED FOR DELIRIUM OR AGITATION IN CANCER PATIENTS

Antipsychotic medications are given to cancer patients to control agitation, sometimes even before prescribers are clear about the cause of the agitation. The most commonly recommended antipsychotic in cancer patients for delirium is haloperidol in low doses. It can be given by mouth (PO), intramuscularly (IM), or intravenously (IV), although it is not routinely given by IV administration in non-cancer patients. Because cancer patients often have low platelet counts, there is concern about giving many IM shots, which can cause bruising and increased pain and discomfort. Other antipsychotics with similar benefits for delirium in cancer patients include the atypical antipsychotics such as olanzapine, quetiapine, ziprasidone, and aripiprazole. Chlorpromazine, which has been available for more than 50 years, is also beneficial. If a patient is agitated and pulling out IV lines or is combative, trying to punch or bite staff, and a less sedating medication such as haloperidol or olanzapine is not effective or able to be given, chlorpromazine can bring on wanted sedation while the medical staff continues attempts to reverse the cause of the delirium and monitors the patient for potential side effects.

Although it is not approved for IV dosing because of the potential to induce cardiac arrhythmias, it is sometimes given IV to someone who is agitated and combative and who is resisting taking oral medications because of the psychotic effects of delirium.

Making Antipsychotics Multitask: The Benefits May Offer Twofers

You may find patients coming to your practice who do not have schizophrenia or bipolar disorder and who have not had a recent delirium, but they are being treated with an antipsychotic medication. Why? For decades, oncologists have appreciated the antiemetic benefits of antipsychotic medications such as prochlorperazine and metoclopramide. In the past decade, studies have demonstrated the antiemetic benefits of a newer, atypical antipsychotic called olanzapine. Not only does this medication work on the dopamine system but also it has some effect on the serotonergic system, which can ease nausea and vomiting. It has been found to be an excellent medication to treat chemotherapy-related nausea.

Olanzapine and another atypical antipsychotic, quetiapine, are sedating (they are considered major tranquilizers). Low nighttime doses of either have been found to help patients sleep better, particularly if their sleep is interrupted by anxiety. As noted in Chapter 2, the atypical antipsychotics can relieve anxiety without the downstream pothole of respiratory depression that can be caused by high-dose benzodiazepines. These medications are best used at low doses for short periods of time when used to treat these non-psychotic symptoms. Unlike the benzodiazepines, the antipsychotics do not carry the side effects of amnesia and disorientation that can lead to falls, so they are commonly used in the inpatient medical setting.

COMMON SIDE EFFECTS OF ANTIPSYCHOTICS

Sedation

Since antipsychotics were developed, even with their robust benefits of resolving psychosis or thought disorders, the side effects have been formidable. The first antipsychotic, chlorpromazine, and medications like it cause sedation. They can have similar anticholinergic side effects as those that occur with the older tricyclic antidepressants as discussed in Chapter 1 (i.e., dry mouth, constipation, urinary retention, blurred vision, weight gain, orthostatic hypotension, and confusion), with the potential for falls, tachycardia, and cardiac conduction abnormalities. Patients often do not like how they feel on these medications because of the side effects, even as their upsetting symptoms of paranoia and auditory hallucinations are resolving.

Dopaminergic Movement Complications

TARDIVE DYSKINESIA

Perhaps the most problematic side effect of the antipsychotic medications is tardive dyskinesia—involuntary muscle movements often of the face, hands, and sometimes trunk. Muscles cannot stay at rest. Cancer patients treated for delirium are usually not on these medications for long periods of time, so tardive dyskinesia is very uncommon, unless a patient had been on the medication years before the cancer and delirium. The newer atypical antipsychotics do not commonly cause this side effect. Recall that this was the side effect that scared Joe so much because his grandmother developed it when she was on chlorpromazine for many years.

AKATHISIA

Akathisia is an internal sense of restlessness that causes patients to pace or move, even while standing in place or lying in bed. This side effect may be relieved with various medications—in a non-delirious patient we might ordinarily give an anticholinergic medication, a benzodiazepine, or a β-blocker such as propranolol to relieve akathisia. But all of these might make a delirium worse. Therefore, lowering the dose of the antipsychotic or changing to a different medication makes sense.

PARKINSONIAN SYMPTOMS

The dopaminergic blockade caused by antipsychotic medications can lead to a clinical picture similar to Parkinson's disease. Antipsychotic medications called high-potency antipsychotics, such as haloperidol, can make patients feel stiff, walk with a stiff festinating gait, have masked facies, or have bilateral or unilateral tremors, making them look and feel as if they have a parkinsonian syndrome.

These symptoms are aggravating and best resolved by lowering dosages or changing antipsychotic medications to a lower potency profile or an atypical antipsychotic. You can detect these symptoms while watching a patient walk into your examination or therapy room. Patients may have trouble showing expression on their faces (masked facies); their gait while walking might appear stiff; and they may have difficulty initiating movements, such as getting up from a chair. They might also have stiffness or rigidity in their arms and wrists, called cogwheeling. Cogwheeling is a ratchet-like click or jerk felt in a joint such as the wrist or elbow with slight rotation. There is resistance, then a little give, and then resistance again, as one might feel with a socket/ratchet wrench. Some say that halo- peridol given by the IV route is less likely to cause extrapyramidal or parkinsonian side effects; however, IV administration of halo- peridol is not allowed in some institutions. We do not expect non- prescribers to check for cogwheeling, but they can recommend that the prescriber do so.

INTRODUCING: MARY

Mary is a 58-year-old woman who was hospitalized for failure
to thrive. She has metastatic lung cancer and has been having
nausea from her chemotherapy. She was referred to you, the
physical therapist, for reconditioning and strengthening. When
you arrive at Mary's room, you find her restless in bed, stating
she feels anxious, but she does not understand why, as she is
feeling better from her nausea and wants to get better. She says
she couldn't wait for you to come, as she wants to get stronger.
She is upset that she got lung cancer even though she never
smoked and is an avid runner, and she is confident she can out-
last the cancer. She cannot believe how awful she feels. When
you examine Mary's strength, you observe that she has a mild
tremor that she did not notice previously. You recall seeing prochlorperazine on her medication list. She says that the medication is new and that it was given to help her nausea. She says the
nausea is much better, but she is more nervous than before.

Mary is likely having a side effect of the antiemetic prochlorperazine called akathisia, a feeling of internal restlessness that is often
accompanied by the inability to relax or sit or stand still. You discuss
this with the primary team and ask if there is a different antiemetic
that Mary might benefit from. She is started on olanzapine, which
helps her nausea and her anxious restlessness.

OTHER SYSTEMIC SIDE EFFECTS OF ANTIPSYCHOTICS

Cardiac and Blood Pressure Effects

As noted with some of the older tricyclic antidepressants, patients on antipsychotic medications can have increased susceptibility to cardiac electric conduction delays and arrhythmias. These arrhythmias (e.g., torsades de pointe), are rare but dangerous. Electrocardiogram monitoring is recommended with higher doses and in those who have pre-existing cardiac risk factors. Clinical logic suggests that as with all prescribed medications, we must balance the potential serious risks of prescribing an antipsychotic to medically vulnerable patients against the serious risks of morbidity and mortality of delirium and the dangers of not prescribing antipsychotics, including serious injury to patients, family, and nurses or the inability to complete medical workups to allow discovery of sources of delirium that can then be treated.

Another cardiovascular side effect is orthostatic hypotension with a subsequent compensatory increase in heart rate. This side effect also occurs with tricyclic antidepressants. Low-potency antipsychotics (e.g., chlorpromazine) can cause sedation and decreased blood pressure. In a physically healthy population—for instance, people who have schizophrenia—this side effect could cause falls and fractures. But in a delirious patient who is already in bed, with nurses monitoring vital signs and patient activity, falls are less likely, unless the patient impulsively struggles to get out of bed.

ANTICHOLINERGIC SIDE EFFECTS

Remember the ditty from Chapter 1 about anticholinergic side effects from head to toe:

Blind as a bat (blurry vision)
Dry as a bone (dry mouth and skin)
The bowel and bladder lose their tone (urinary retention and constipation)
And the heart runs alone (tachycardia)
Hot as a hare (feverish)
Red as a beet (flushing)
Mad as a hatter (hallucinations)

IT IS IMPORTANT TO INFORM PATIENTS (OR FAMILY MEMBERS) ABOUT REACTIONS BEFORE THEY OCCUR

When patients are receiving antipsychotics in the cancer setting, it is usually for delirium. When a patient is not attending to reality or they are having fluctuations in their alertness, it is difficult to explain to them the potential side effects of medications. But we have been in situations in which explanations to family or friends can be helpful. As a non-prescriber, you can inform the patient or family how mild sedation can be beneficial, even if it will not correct a reversed sleep–wake cycle of delirium. Explaining the possibility of unwanted reactions such as increased anxiety or akathisia can help a patient or family know what to look out for. Informing the patient or family why doctors or nurses may examine the patient's limbs for stiffness or tremors can be an opportunity to discuss the goals of antipsychotic treatment in these situations and affirm that the medical caregivers know what to watch for with regard to negative effects.

NEUROLEPTIC MALIGNANT SYNDROME

Neuroleptic malignant syndrome (NMS) is an extremely rare side effect of the older antipsychotics caused by a severe decrease in dopamine activity. It can occur at any dose of an antipsychotic, and after any length of duration of treatment. It is life-threatening and demands cessation of the antipsychotic and referral for close medical monitoring, usually in an ICU setting. Symptoms of NMS include fever, muscle rigidity (cogwheeling), and confusion, along with abnormal metabolic factors such as unstable vital signs (blood pressure and heart rate), increased white blood cell count, increased creatine phosphokinase, and myoglobin in the urine. The non-prescriber may only hear about the patient feeling feverish or stiff. When the non-prescriber becomes aware that the patient is taking an antipsychotic, the non-prescriber can advocate notifying the patient's prescriber. Prescribers can measure prolactin levels over time to ensure they are declining after cessation of the antipsychotic medication. Sometimes patients receive muscle relaxants such as baclofen or dopamine agonists such as bromocriptine to improve symptomatic rigidity.

Atypical antipsychotics are considered much safer than the older, traditional antipsychotics. Tardive dyskinesia, extrapyramidal symptoms, and NMS are rare with atypical antipsychotics; however, prescribers are concerned about long-term side effects such as glucose abnormalities, lipid anomalies, weight gain, and cardiac

Box 3.9 SIDE EFFECTS OF ATYPICAL ANTIPSYCHOTICS

- Metabolic syndrome
  - Hyperglycemia
  - Hyperlipidemia
  - Weight gain
- QTc prolongation

conduction delays with vulnerable patients and with longer term use, as noted in Box 3.9.

Extrapyramidal side effects and akathisia are possible with atypical antipsychotics. However, they are more rare than with most of the more traditional antipsychotics (except risperidone).

SAFETY CONSIDERATIONS—REMEMBER POTENTIAL CONTRAINDICATIONS

Given the many potential side effects of antipsychotic medications, it is difficult to be aware of all potential contraindications. When cancer patients are seeing many specialists, it can be very helpful for the non-prescriber to be aware of the medical issues of their patients and, if necessary, be another resource of protection by having important information at their fingertips and open communication lines to prescribers.

If a delirious patient has a cardiac condition such as atrial fibrillation, cardiology may be consulted to ensure the patient can tolerate any medications that might prolong their cardiac conduction, which would be measured by the QTc.

If delirium occurs in a patient with parkinsonism, the non-prescriber can advocate to avoid antipsychotics that might readily worsen that syndrome (haloperidol and risperidone). Prescribers may consider antipsychotics such as quetiapine or clozapine if available, and consult neurology if needed.

If a patient has diabetes or glucose abnormalities and needs to receive an atypical antipsychotic such as olanzapine or quetiapine, it is recommended that they be used for short periods and glucose be monitored regularly. These recommendations are similar for diabetics who need to receive steroids for extended periods of time. Consultation with an endocrinologist may be useful.

As with the older antidepressants that can have anticholinergic side effects, prescribers should be hesitant to use medications such as chlorpromazine or even olanzapine or quetiapine in patients who already have urinary retention or severe constipation. Although these side effects may seem like nothing more than a nuisance to the patient, the non-prescriber should encourage the patient to report these symptoms to their prescribers.

Many of the side effects that antipsychotics can cause if used alone may be exacerbated when combined with other medications, either because of drug interactions that adversely impact metabolism of one of the medications or because of a synergistic combined consequence.

Drug Interactions

As with all medications, the potential for drug interactions with other medications must be considered. Table 3.4 highlights potential drug interactions in the cancer setting when antipsychotics are given with other medications.

Table 3.4 Impact of Drug Interactions and Combinations
with Antipsychotics

Antipsychotic + antiemetic (prochlorperazine/metoclopramide) =

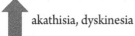 akathisia, dyskinesia

Antipsychotic + methadone or ondansetron =

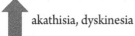 likelihood of QTc prolongation and serious arrhythmia

Antipsychotic + benzodiazepine or an antihistamine = sedation

Traditional antipsychotic + some antidepressants = parkinsonism

---

HOW PSYCHO-ONCOLOGY PRESCRIBERS CHOOSE AN ANTIPSYCHOTIC

The following algorithm provides clues about choosing anti-psychotics in the setting of delirium and cancer:

Not agitated, or hypoactive (difficult to arouse):
    Low-dose haloperidol PO or IV, titrated as needed
Monitor for parkinsonism, akathisia, QTc, sedation

If agitated, hyperactive (restless or combative):
    Haloperidol with lorazepam, titrated as needed
Monitor for parkinsonism, QTc, oversedation
OR

Olanzapine or quetiapine taken at bedtime or twice a day
(These medications are given orally and need to be swallowed—not indicated for patients who cannot take medications by mouth or cannot swallow)
Monitor for QTc and daytime sedation

OR

Chlorpromazine, either PO, IM, or IV, is helpful for very agitated, combative patients
Monitor for QTc, blood pressure and pulse, sedation, anticholinergic side effects

As discussed previously, long-term side effects of antipsychotics, such as tardive dyskinesia, that were seen with chronic use in people with schizophrenia or bipolar disorder are rare in medically ill patients because they are taken off antipsychotics as their delirium resolves. But when families research these medications on the internet, they are likely to obtain information that may or may not be appropriate to the current situation. It is better to inform people up front what they will read about, rather than having to be defensive afterwards.

ALTERNATIVE MEDICATIONS FOR AGITATION

When patients cannot tolerate antipsychotic medications and they continue to be agitated or combative, mood stabilizers that are often used to treat manic episodes may be helpful. They can be sedating, and some can be given IV for patients who cannot take oral medications, or who are too agitated to take oral medications.

Depot antipsychotic medications are given by injection, yielding a slow, continual release of the medication over weeks to months.

They are used to improve adherence among people with schizophrenia or bipolar disorder. In general, having a patient take a medication once every few weeks or months is easier than getting them to take the medication daily. However, psychiatric depot medications are not generally used in the cancer population because of potentially fast changes in medical status due to the cancer or cancer treatment and the potential need to stop all nonvital medications quickly.

DELIRIUM AT THE END OF LIFE

There is controversy about whether to treat the symptoms of delirium, such as hallucinations or paranoia or confusion, which occur toward the end of life (terminal delirium). Because delirium is viewed as a natural part of the dying process, some argue that it should not be treated. They may also be concerned that the medications can cause sedation at a time when family or friends might want to engage with the dying person at the end of their life. Others believe that the psychotic symptoms should be treated because these symptoms can become frightening and upsetting and the dying person may not be able to communicate their fear and upset.

It is important to recall that the goal of treating delirium in someone who is not dying is to reverse the etiology of the delirium; symptom control with the antipsychotic is important to facilitate that. In the patient who is dying, the goal is to control the symptoms and ease suffering.

SUMMARY

Antipsychotics are an important class of medications used to treat the symptoms of delirium. Antipsychotics treat psychosis, agitation, confusion, insomnia, anxiety, as well as nausea in the cancer setting. Because antipsychotics are commonly used to treat primary psychotic psychiatric disorders such as schizophrenia and bipolar disorder, they may frighten patients and family members when used in the cancer setting. However, it must be remembered that the symptoms of delirium are also frightening and dangerous. Awareness of the pearls and potholes of antipsychotic treatment can help non-prescribers be an important source of information, education, communication, and support for their patients, families, and other members of the oncology treatment team.

NOTES

1. American Psychiatric Association (2010).
2. Lonergan E, Britton AE, Luxenberg J, Wyller T. Antipsychotics for delirium. *Cochrane Database Syst Rev.* 2007;2007(2):CD005594.
3. Burry L, Mehta S, Perreault MM, et al. Antipsychotics for treatment of delirium in hospitalized non-ICU patients. *Cochrane Database Syst Rev.* 2018;2018(6):CD005594.
4. Breitbart W, Marotta R, Platt MM et al. A double-blind trial of haloperidol, chlorpromazine, and lorazepam in the treatment of delirium in hospitalized AIDS patients. *Am J Psychiatry.* 1996 Feb;153(2):231–237. doi:10.1176/ajp.153.2.231.

Chapter 4

Medications for Sleep Disturbance

INTRODUCTION

Sleep disorders have been reported in up to 75% of newly diagnosed or recently treated cancer patients.[1] Although about one-third of all adults report sleep disturbances, less than 15% meet criteria for a sleep disorder.[2]

Formal sleep disorders last at least three nights per week and last longer than three months in otherwise healthy adults. Inadequate or too much sleep can impair medical and emotional well-being, daytime functioning, and cognitive alertness and can lead to anxiety or depression. Insomnia, or sleep disturbance, manifests in many ways in people with cancer. Usually we think of sleep disorders in terms of difficulty falling asleep or staying asleep despite having adequate opportunity to sleep. Although this chapter focuses primarily on those who have trouble getting to or staying asleep, there are also people with cancer who have hypersomnia—they sleep too much. Sleep complaints may be intermittent, often related to specific situations or medical problems, but can also develop into an ongoing syndrome. Some patients will sleep but do not have restful sleep because of pre-existing disorders such as sleep apnea. Non-prescribers are often called upon to assist with teaching healthy nonpharmacologic sleep hygiene techniques. However, it is important to recognize when a proper medication can assist or supplement good sleep habits. We discuss the potential benefits and pitfalls of medications used to induce and maintain sleep and how patients can integrate medication use into the standard nonmedicinal sleep-promoting techniques. You will be able to monitor for potential side effects of hypnotics (sleep medications), including cognitive and balance abnormalities, as well as compromised daytime energy and alertness, which might keep patients from taking these medications altogether.

AVOIDING THE POTHOLES OF SLEEP DISTURBANCE DIAGNOSIS IN CANCER PATIENTS

Sleep disorders can involve difficulty falling asleep, difficulty staying asleep because of nighttime awakenings, or early morning awakening. Formal sleep disorders are often determined by objective observation in sleep laboratories, although subjective feelings about sleep quality are important to ascertain, especially in people with cancer, who have multiple potential causes of not falling or staying asleep at night. Sleep studies that monitor brain activity, eye movements, and muscle tone measure sleep and wake cycles. This type of elaborate testing is often not feasible in someone with cancer who likely has already undergone many procedures and spent much time away from home. There are now home study kits that may be more easily used by cancer patients. A major sleep problem is not only based on how frequently it occurs but also when it has a negative consequential impact on the quality of a person's life socially, occupationally, medically, behaviorally, or in some other important area of functioning.

Sleep is divided into two phases: rapid eye movement (REM) or dream sleep and non-REM (NREM) sleep. People are behaviorally less activated during REM sleep, although their brains show wakefulness and activated brain wave monitoring. A common pattern for sleeping is to move from shallow stages of NREM sleep to deeper stages and then into REM sleep. Each complete cycle usually lasts 90–120 minutes. Dream phases, which encompass approximately one-fourth of sleep time, last longer and NREM phases become shorter as the night progresses. In people with cancer, sleep–wake cycles can be impaired for many reasons. Thus, when a patient tells you or a prescriber "I can't sleep," clarifying this statement by considering the features of sleep disturbances noted in Box 4.1 can help pinpoint the reason for the impairment.

Box 4.1 FEATURES OF SLEEP COMPLAINTS

- Difficulty falling asleep
  - How long does it take to fall asleep?
    - Might there be any medical or medication explanations?
    - Do you feel wide awake at night?
    - Do you have endless worry or thinking about problems?
- Nighttime awakenings, either with ease or difficulty falling back asleep
  - How many times do you wake up at night after falling asleep?
    - For what reason: urination, pain, hot flashes, cough?
  - How long does it take you to fall back asleep?
- Early morning awakening
  - How early do you wake up for the last time in the morning?
  - Do you feel refreshed?
    - How long does it take after awakening to feel fully alert?

RISK FACTORS FOR SLEEP DISTURBANCE IN CANCER PATIENTS

The barriers to a good night's sleep can be chronic, having begun in a person's life long before a cancer diagnosis, or may be related to severe anxiety, thought ruminations, obsessions, depression, or physical symptoms or may be secondary to side effects of medications. Sleep disturbances may even be related to the biological aspects of the cancer or cancer treatment, such as inflammatory processes. Other risk factors may include older age and changing sleep patterns, female gender (especially postmenopausal), family and personal history of sleep disturbances, and a predilection to becoming hyperaroused. In addition, an increased need to urinate, gastric upset, and other physical symptoms such as coughing and shortness of breath can impair sleep. Other factors that can exacerbate sleep disturbances include excessive daytime naps or time in bed, poor sleep hygiene, and unrealistic sleep expectations.

Predisposing factors for sleep disturbance are noted in Boxes 4.2 and 4.3. They include stress; hot flashes; hospitalization (a hospital

---

Box 4.2 PREDISPOSING FACTORS THAT MAY PRECLUDE SLEEP
IN CANCER PATIENTS

- Changing sleep patterns of aging
- Chronic sleep disturbance
- Light sleepers who are easily aroused
- History of night work shift sleeping patterns
- Family history of sleep disturbances
- Sleep apnea

Box 4.3 FACTORS INFLUENCING SLEEP PROBLEMS IN PEOPLE
WITH CANCER

- Stress, uncertainty, seeing little hope for change
- Hot flashes (in menopausal women and in men on androgen deprivation therapy)
- Hospitalization
- Radiation therapy
- Pain syndromes
- Anxiety or restlessness
- Worry ruminations or obsessiveness
- Depression causing too little or too much sleep
- Other physical distress (i.e., cough, shortness of breath, gastric upset, headaches, urinary frequency)
- Medications (i.e., corticosteroids, other hormonal agents, activating agents)
  - Feeling wide awake at night
- Biological aspects of the cancer (inflammatory processes)
- Unrealistic sleep expectations
- Too much daytime napping
- Substances that either activate (i.e., caffeine) or sedate then activate (i.e., alcohol)

---

is not necessarily the best place for rest and relaxation); radiation therapy; medications such as corticosteroids, hormonal agents, and stimulants; and various cancer treatments. Pain syndromes can either keep people awake at night or make nighttime trips to the bathroom more treacherous. Other medical causes of sleep problems include thyroid dysfunction and substance use, intoxication, or withdrawal (alcohol and other drugs). Anemia can lead to fatigue and excessive sleeping. Some patients may be retired from jobs in which they worked at night and slept during the day. They can have difficulty trying to adjust to a hospital routine or cancer patient routine that rewards sleep during the night and wakefulness during the day.

ASK, BECAUSE THEY MAY NOT TELL; TELL BEFORE THEY ASK

In cancer patients, sleep disorders often occur along with pain syndromes or other physical problems and therefore may have no clear patterns. As previously discussed with regard to anxiety and depressive syndromes in cancer patients, sleep problems may also be common after a new diagnosis, after a crisis such as a cancer recurrence or learning that a treatment did not work, or when physical symptoms worsen or do not get better. Although sleep will usually improve after these crises, sleep architecture does not always return to patients' pre-cancer baseline. Sleep problems are highly prevalent in people with advanced cancer, especially when they have significant physical symptoms, as noted in Box 4.4. However, instead of a focus on predisposing factors, sleep complaints are often diagnosed as sleep disorders. If you do not ask the patient about their particular nuances of sleep, they may not recognize what is important to tell.

The impact of not sleeping well, as highlighted in Box 4.5, includes both physical and emotional consequences including compromised daytime energy, poor concentration, mood, and anxiety changes, as

Box 4.4 MEDICAL LOOK-ALIKES FOR SLEEP DISTURBANCE

- Pain, cough, urinary or bowel frequency, hot flashes
- Hormonal imbalances (i.e., thyroid dysfunction)
- Anemia leading to fatigue and excessive sleep
- Substance use, intoxication, or withdrawal
- Medications: steroids, stimulants, antidepressants, delirium, mania
- Sleep apnea or other breathing difficulties
- Restless legs

well as potentially worsened pain and other medical issues, such as cardiovascular health and diabetes control. Cognitive functioning and decision-making capabilities may also be impaired, and there may be a higher likelihood of falls and accidents.

Box 4.5 POSSIBLE IMPACT OF SLEEP DISTURBANCES

- Decreased energy
- Poor concentration or attention
- More complaints of forgetfulness
- Lower mood
- Increased anxiety
- More physical complaints and potential compromise of other medical issues
- Subjective feeling of poor decision-making
- Increased risk of falls and accidents

Unfortunately, most patients will not readily include sleep disturbance in their list of complaints to their oncology teams. The non-prescriber is an important advocate to encourage this discussion with all providers. Asking patients about their sleep habits, as well as how long it takes to fall asleep and how often they wake up in the middle of the night, helps patients clarify these issues and encourages them to address the problems with their prescribers, as noted in Box 4.6. Although you are not the sleep

---

Box 4.6 QUESTIONS YOU CAN ASK TO CLARIFY SLEEP
DISTURBANCES

How often do you nap during the day? How long each time?

Do you have regular sleep and wake times?

What time do you go to sleep?

Are you afraid to close your eyes at night for fear that you will die in your sleep?

Do you find yourself worrying about the next diagnostic test, or the results of that test weeks in advance?

When do you wake up? How many times?

How long does it take you to fall back asleep?

Do you have pain or urinary or bowel problems that interfere with sleep?

Are there other physical symptoms that might interfere with sleep (i.e., coughing, nausea, or breathing problems)?

Do you have restless legs?

Are the sleep problems ongoing or sporadic? Situation-specific or generalized?

Are your sleep problems chronic or new with the cancer?

Are your sleep problems related to recent (lifestyle) changes?
Tobacco cessation; decrease or increase in smoking
Alcohol cessation; decrease or increase in drinking
Other substance use (e.g., marijuana, supplements)
Or recent cessation, decrease, or increase in substance use
Is your sleep difficulty interfering with your ability to carry on and enjoy life?
How difficult is it for you to get up in the morning?
When is the last time you can remember having a "good" sleep at night where you felt refreshed in the morning?
Have you been told you have sleep apnea? Do you have a machine to help with that?
Do you use your sleep apnea machine?

expert, asking patients about snoring, daytime fatigue, and a history of high blood pressure may assist in a diagnosis of sleep apnea that may have been overlooked. By asking about sleep habits, especially in the presence of the patient's partner, you might also hear about other syndromes, such as restless legs syndrome, or other sleep problems, such as sleepwalking or agitation during sleep.

The algorithm presented next can help you understand a patient's sleep disturbance and what remedies might be appropriate for that person.

ALGORITHM FOR DIAGNOSING SLEEP DISTURBANCE IN CANCER PATIENTS

If there is a personal or family history of sleep disorder or abnormal sleep patterns?

OR

Potential medical or physical causes of difficulty falling asleep or staying asleep have been addressed sufficiently (recent onset of sleep difficulties with new physical complaints or prescription of new medications).

AND

The patient consistently has trouble falling asleep or staying asleep

AND

The patient is NOT feeling rested upon awakening?

OR

The patient is sleeping too much or not active enough during daytime hours?

AND

There is *not* a diagnosis of depression or an anxiety disorder that better explains the sleep complaints as part of a larger syndrome?

=

Consider a sleep disturbance that may be addressed by sleep hygiene techniques, a sleep medication, or addressing specific physical instigators or causes.

INTERVENTIONS FOR SLEEP PROBLEMS

Non-prescribers and prescribers can review nonpharmacologic interventions for sleep problems with patients prior to, or concurrent with, a pharmacologic approach. We do not review the sleep hygiene techniques in detail here, but they are listed in Box 4.7.

Sleep hygiene techniques, which might include using relaxation techniques, progressive muscle relaxation and visual imagery, and the core of cognitive–behavioral therapy for insomnia can often obviate the need for sleep medications. These educational and practical strategies have been found to decrease the time required to fall asleep and increase total sleep time and improve quality of life.

Box 4.7 SLEEP HYGIENE TECHNIQUES

- Proper environment
  - The bedroom is for sleep.
  - Set times for going to sleep and waking.
  - Limit nap times and time in bed that is not for sleep.
  - Exercise regularly, but not too late in the day.
  - Avoid caffeine or late-day wakefulness agents.
  - Avoid alcohol before bedtime.
  - Avoid clock watching.
  - Avoid any screen time if you are going to sleep in bed.
  - Change tablet screen mode to "night shift."
- Relaxation techniques
  - Abdominal breathing
  - Mindfulness meditation
  - Visual imagery
  - Square technique
- Cognitive techniques—Keep paper and pen next to bed for downloading thoughts.

- Avoid catastrophizing thinking.
- Avoid forecasting.
- Avoid making comparisons with others or your past experiences.
- Comfort foods
  - Consider protein *plus* glucose if patient can tolerate.
  - Consider tryptophan-rich foods (turkey).

WHETHER THE SYMPTOMS OF INSOMNIA WILL TIP A PRESCRIBER TO SUGGEST A SLEEP MEDICATION

If the nonpharmacologic sleep hygiene methods are insufficient to bring on consistent restful sleep, or the patient is not able to apply them consistently, the following medication options may be tried. However, it is useful for the non-prescriber to continue to encourage the nonmedicinal strategies so the medications may be able to work at the lowest effective doses and for the shortest amount of time necessary. Recommendations suggest sleep medications be given for no longer than 1 month; unfortunately, as with other psychopharmacology in cancer patients, there is no one-size-fits-all norm. Reassessment for sleep medications should be ongoing, with changes made as circumstances for each patient change. Both the prescriber and the non-prescriber can keep sleep hygiene and sleep medications on their radar screen, even though neither may be a sleep expert.

MEDS FOR HEADS

Understanding the Strategies of the Psycho-Oncology Medication Prescriber

OVERVIEW OF THE MEDS—JUST GET FAMILIAR WITH THE NAMES

Over-the-counter (OTC) medications
  Diphenhydramine (Benadryl)
  Melatonin
Z drugs
  Zolpidem (Ambien)
  Zaleplon (Sonata)
  Eszopiclone (Lunesta)
Benzodiazepines for sleep
  Temazepam (Restoril)
  Lorazepam (Ativan)
  Clonazepam (Klonopin)
  Diazepam (Valium)
Melatonin receptor agonists
  Ramelteon (Rozerem)
  Tasimelteon (Hetlioz)
Sedating antidepressants used to initiate sleep
  Doxepin (Sinequan)
  Mirtazapine (Remeron)
  Amitriptyline (Elavil)
Antipsychotics
  Olanzapine (Zyprexa)

Quetiapine (Seroquel)
Orexin receptor antagonists
Suvorexant (Belsomra)
Cannabinoids

CASE: SAMANTHA

Samantha is a 49-year-old woman with noninvasive bladder cancer. After a transurethral resection of the bladder tumor, she has been getting bacillus Calmette–Guérin (BCG) immuno-therapy treatments every 6 weeks.

She has been having increasing difficulty falling asleep. In her psychotherapy sessions with you, she denies obvious anx-iety but finds herself staying up at night reading about bladder cancer prognosis and treatment, and blogs of those who have had bladder cancer. She is getting more fatigued during the day and has more difficulty focusing on her job as an administra-tive assistant. She wonders if her fatigue is related to her BCG treatments or from not sleeping. As far as you know, she has been otherwise healthy. She has taken zolpidem periodically in the past for long airplane flights. You suggest she speak with her pri-mary care doctor or oncologist about what might be causing her fatigue and ask about getting a prescription for zolpidem. In the meantime, you continue to reinforce sleep hygiene techniques with her.

The essence of a good sleep medication is to be sedating, quickly. However, if it works very quickly, a patient needs to know this so they do not fall asleep sitting in the bathroom or at the kitchen table. The ideal sleep medication should have effective activity to match a normal night's sleep—approximately 8 hours. It should not leave a patient wide awake at 4 am or leave a patient with a groggy hangover feeling on awakening in the morning; additionally, it should not compromise a person's thinking or physical coordination the day after taking it. The medication should not interact with any of the patient's other medications and should not have negative effects on other organs/systems of the patient—(i.e., liver, kidneys, neurological or cardiovascular systems). It should also not cause any urinary or bowel problems while a patient is sleeping.

The common sleep medications are classified into eight major categories: OTC medications of antihistamines and melatonin; melatonin receptor agonists; cannabinoids; and traditional sleep-inducing prescription medications—Z drugs (non-benzodiazepine hypnotics), benzodiazepines, sedating antidepressants, major tranquilizers or antipsychotics, and sedating antiseizure medications.

MYTHS THAT KEEP PATIENTS FROM TAKING SLEEP MEDICATIONS

The widespread use of the non-benzodiazepine hypnotics (Z drugs) for inducing sleep has in part been related to patients having less fear of addiction from them. In the past decade, with wider use of these medications for longer periods of time, we have become aware of individual susceptibility to the dependence, tolerance, and addictive consequences of these medications. Their popularity in part is due to the known negative impact of the benzodiazepines and, before them, the barbiturates, which are highly addictive medications used for inducing sleep. Prescribers often will ask patients, "If you are not getting good sleep every single night, would you be willing to accept one good night out of two or three?" Many people will say "Sure." Then they are directed to take the sleep medications sporadically, obviating the downstream potential of dependence or tolerance.

THE MEDESCORT GUIDE TO TREAT SLEEP DISTURBANCES

How Sleep Medications Work, and Why It Is Important for Non-Prescribers and Their Patients to Know About This

OVER-THE-COUNTER MEDICATIONS FOR SLEEP

Antihistamines

Most OTC sleep-enhancing medications have an antihistamine-like chemistry. These medications are often found in antiallergy formulations and can have sedative effects—which induce sleep. Sleep may come more quickly and there may be lasting influence throughout the night. The side effects of these medications when used as sleep aides include morning grogginess ("hangover" effect) as well as daytime sedation; weight gain and anticholinergic side effects such as those previously discussed with regard to antidepressant and antipsychotic medications—dry mouth, urinary retention, constipation, and confusion, which are even more pronounced in the elderly.

Melatonin

Melatonin is a hormone found naturally in the body that helps adjust the body's internal sleep–wake cycles. Darkness causes the body to produce more melatonin, which signals the body to prepare for sleep. Light decreases melatonin production and signals the body to prepare for being awake. Some people who have trouble sleeping have low levels of melatonin. Studies are mixed on how well melatonin works to help induce sleep. To help insomnia, melatonin is taken 30–60 minutes prior to bedtime. It may be beneficial to take melatonin a few hours prior to sleep to help with delayed sleep phase syndrome, where a person's ability to fall asleep is delayed beyond what is acceptable. Melatonin may also assist with adjusting to jet lag with improvement in alertness and body movement, although it may not help with inducing sleep when jet lagged. Because this is a supplement, it is important to use products vetted by the U.S. Pharmacopeia organization.

Dosing ranges from 0.3 to 5 mg at bedtime. Adverse reactions are usually not serious, although any sleep medication can cause morning or daytime grogginess. It is useful to ensure there are no drug–drug interactions with other medications patients are taking, such as anticoagulants, anticonvulsants, blood pressure medications, and diabetes medications.

PRESCRIPTION MEDICATIONS USED FOR SLEEP
The Z Drugs
Zolpidem, zopiclone, and (es)zaleplon, also known as Z drugs, are non-benzodiazepine hypnotics with minimal anxiolytic effect and lower risk for tolerance and dependence. They are listed in Table 4.1. They really are like "knockout" drugs. Zolpidem has been known to help patients get to sleep (very quickly), but not all patients stay asleep for 7 or more hours. In those situations, trials of controlled-release zolpidem have been found to be helpful. Some patients get an unusual, unpleasant, or metallic taste in their mouths with eszopiclone.

Table 4.1 The Z Drugs[a]

Generic Name	Brand Name	Starting Dose
Zolpidem	Ambien	2.5–10 mg bedtime
Zaleplon	Sonata	5–10 mg bedtime
Eszopiclone	Lunesta	1–3 mg bedtime (some get a metallic taste)

[a]All have rapid action and increase sleep duration.

Hypnotics have potential side effects including early morning awakening, hangover effect, and daytime grogginess. Other common side effects include dizziness, headache, and nausea. They should not be used daily for more than 1 month at a time. In addition, these medications have been rarely noted to cause hallucinations, confusion, and short-term memory loss.

Benzodiazepines

Benzodiazepines, such as lorazepam, temazepam, and clonazepam, are frequently prescribed sleep medications for those experiencing acute crises. They are listed in Table 4.2. Long-term use can cause dependence and tolerance and loss of efficacy, as described in Chapter 2. The benzodiazepines relieve insomnia. Unlike the Z drugs, most will also treat anxiety that causes a patient to have difficulty inducing or maintaining sleep. There is a risk of too much sedation with all sleep medications if the patient concurrently uses alcohol; has hepatic or kidney disease (because of impaired clearing of the medication); pulmonary disease (because benzodiazepines can suppress respirations) or sleep apnea; or is taking another medication that causes central nervous system depression, such as opioids or antiseizure medications.

Table 4.2 Benzodiazepines Used for Sleep Disturbance

Generic Name	Brand Name	Starting Dose	Non-Psychiatrist Sky View Focus
Temazepam	Restoril	7.5–30 mg	Shorter onset Reduces sleep latency Increases sleep duration Does not treat anxiety
Clonazepam	Klonopin	0.25–1 mg	Long acting Reduces sleep fragmentation Helps anxiety and panic
Lorazepam	Ativan	0.5–1 mg	Intermediate onset Reduces sleep latency Helps anxiety
Alprazolam	Xanax	0.25–1 mg	Fast onset Reduces sleep latency Helps anxiety and panic Intermediate acting with abrupt end of action—benefits may not last the night

CASE: SAM

Sam is a 56-year-old man with non-Hodgkin's lymphoma who has had chemotherapy. He comes to see you for his rehabilitation therapy session to help with various strengthening and mobility limitations since his treatment. He notes that he falls asleep easily but wakes up at approximately 2 a.m. and has difficulty getting back to sleep despite trying meditation and other sleep hygiene techniques. He stopped smoking tobacco when he was diagnosed with his cancer, and he relates that cigarettes always used to calm him down if he awoke in the night. He never used alcohol. His primary care doctor started trazodone, but it made his dry mouth worse, as did the OTC antihistamines he tried before that. He said he had tried melatonin in the past, but it did not work for him. When he tried alprazolam, he woke up after a few hours. Sam is cognitively sharp. You provide him with psychoeducation that reiterates that nicotine is a stimulant that interrupts sleep, although it may provide some mood-stabilizing effects for some people. You suggest he speak with his prescriber about trying another medication to help his sleep, and you tell him that you can speak with his oncologist as well. When you speak with his prescriber, you describe the sleep hygiene techniques and medications Sam has already tried and ask whether a short course of temazepam or clonazepam, which are longer acting benzodiazepines, might be helpful for Sam.

ADDITIONAL MEDICATIONS USED FOR INSOMNIA

There are other classes of medications listed in Table 4.3 that are not indicated primarily for sleep but that are used for their sedating properties to induce or maintain sleep. These medications

Table 4.3 Additional Medications Used for Insomnia
in Cancer Patients

Medication	Starting Dose
Sedating Antidepressants	
Trazodone (Desyrel), heterocyclic	25–100 mg bedtime
Doxepin (Sinequan), tricyclic	10–50 mg bedtime
Mirtazapine (Remeron), tetracyclic	7.5–15 mg bedtime
Amitriptyline (Elavil), tricyclic	10–50 mg bedtime
Nortriptyline (Pamelor), tricyclic	10–50 mg bedtime
Atypical Antipsychotic/Mood Stabilizers	
Olanzapine (Zyprexa)	2.5–5 mg bedtime
Quetiapine (Seroquel)	25–50 mg bedtime
Lurasidone (Latuda)	20–40 mg bedtime
Melatonin Receptor Agonist	
Ramelteon (Rozerem)	8 mg bedtime
Antiseizure Medications	
Gabapentin (Neurontin)	100–300 mg bedtime
Pregabalin (Lyrica)	25–50 mg bedtime

include antidepressants, atypical antipsychotics, melatonin, and medications in the antiepileptic class.

Antidepressants

Antidepressants have been useful for sleep disorders. This is particularly true if the sleep difficulty is related to a major depressive episode—if the depression does not get treated, the sleep symptoms may be treated symptomatically but will not resolve until the depression is resolved. Even if there is no depressive syndrome, sedating antidepressants can help induce sleep. These medications include trazodone, mirtazapine, amitriptyline, and doxepin. Trazodone is primarily serotonergic and, due to daytime sedation, may not be tolerated well in the high doses needed to treat depression; however, 25–100 mg at bedtime may be sufficient for sleep. Side effects include loss of appetite, dry mouth, and constipation. A rare but uncomfortable side effect in men is priapism, a prolonged and painful erection that does not resolve following ejaculation. The veins of the penis are abnormally narrowed so extra blood that enters the penis to produce an erection cannot exit normally and the organ remains engorged and painful. Patients should apply ice and go to an emergency room for draining of the blood.

Mirtazapine's chemical nature mimics antihistaminic effects at lower doses. The resulting sedating effects of mirtazapine induce sleep. Some believe that the antihistaminic chemistry of mirtazapine is relatively more potent at lower doses compared to its antidepressant effect. It has no gastric side effects and is usually well tolerated. When used for sleeping, it is taken on an as-needed basis. Similarly, the tricyclic medications amitriptyline and doxepin have chemical structures that induce antihistaminic effects, causing sedation and inducing sleep. However, these medications have anticholinergic side effects that can cause confusion and other problems noted previously.

All medications that induce sedation can lead to falls if the patient wakes up at night. Placing night lights along the path from the bedroom to the bathroom, kitchen, or living room may prevent falls if a patient awakens to urinate, get something to eat, get a pain medication, or go read in another room.

Atypical Antipsychotics

The atypical antipsychotics discussed in detail in Chapter 3 are also used to induce and maintain sleep. Olanzapine and quetiapine may have antihistaminic, anticholinergic, or serotonergic effects that help induce sleep and are used when anxiety accompanies the sleep disturbance and when the patient cannot tolerate a Z drug or a benzodiazepine because of adverse side effects (e.g., respiratory dysfunction or confusion). These medications help counter the agitating effects of steroids given as part of a cancer treatment regimen. Lurasidone is another atypical antipsychotic used for this purpose. Risperidone is also an atypical antipsychotic that might reduce anxiety; however, it does not usually have significant hypnotic effects and thus does not induce sleep.

CASE: GEORGE

George is a 71-year-old man with prostate cancer. He has been undergoing androgen deprivation therapy (ADT). He has been seeing you for relationship issues because he has been arguing with his husband more often and, because of the ADT, they are no longer able to have sex, which had always been pleasurable and an automatic connection for them. He also reports that his anger is worse later in the day when he is more fatigued; however, he has been having trouble falling asleep. You have been working with George on anger management and sleep hygiene strategies, but they have not been helpful. You think about speaking with his oncologist or nurse practitioiner about considering either a benzodiazepine, a sedating antidepressant such as mirtazapine, or a sedating antipsychotic such as olanzapine. You recall that although George has been sober for 10 years, he had been alcohol dependent, so you think a benzodiazepine may not be the best first choice. George's nurse practitioner decides to first try a low dose of mirtazapine at night to help George sleep better and decrease his irritability.

Melatonin Receptor Agonists

Ramelteon is a selective melatonin receptor agonist. It enhances sleep through effects on sleep regulatory mechanisms in the brain rather than inducing a groggy feeling. Ramelteon binds to melatonin receptors and decreases the evening alerting signal to enhance sleep onset, and it ultimately helps reinforce or shift the timing of the circadian system. Some patients may find that their sleep continues to improve over a few weeks as the circadian rhythm is restored. Side effects include liver dysfunction. As with other medications, drug–drug interactions should be considered. Ramelteon does not seem to induce sleep very successfully for many patients. Some believe that it needs to be taken over a period of time to change the physiology of a person's sleep pattern and have a positive effect on sleep. It has been used to try to recalibrate the sleep cycles of patients who are delirious and not sleeping at night. It is often used in these patients in conjunction with antipsychotics.

Antiepileptic Medications

The antiseizure medications, gabapentin and pregabalin, that are used for anxiety are sometimes prescribed for insomnia as well. In the cancer setting, they are most often used for neuropathic pain. Their sedating quality and anxiolytic properties make them helpful for resistant sleep problems. Because gabapentin has been found to relieve hot flashes, it may be very helpful for patients whose sleep is disturbed periodically through the night by hot flashes and anxiety that are induced by menopause in women or ADT medications in men with prostate cancer.

A NEW CLASS OF SLEEP MEDICATION (SUVOREXANT)

Suvorexant (Belsomra) is a relatively new sleep medication that does not work on the γ-aminobutyric acid receptor system as do the benzodiazepines and the Z drugs. It is an orexin inhibitor. Orexin is a peptide released from the hypothalamus that helps maintain wakefulness. Medications such as modafinil and armodafinil help people fight fatigue and sedation during the day. Suvorexant helps prevent arousal and induces sleep. Common side effects include drowsiness, dizziness, headache, unusual dreams, dry mouth, cough, and diarrhea. Suvorexant can interact with medications that are CYP3A4 inhibitors, so communication with the prescriber about possible interactions with medications such as ketoconazole, erythromycin, fluconazole, ritonavir, and others may be welcome. Online tables provide more information about the potential interactions.

An Old Solution for Sleep and Anxiety Makes a Comeback

CANNABIS

The popularity of cannabis has led people with cancer to try it for many symptoms, including nausea, pain, low appetite, and anxiety, as well as insomnia. In part due to the dissimilar and changing legalization status in different locales in the United States, the quality and effects of cannabis are irregular, although they are becoming more standardized as the cannabis industry grows and medical marijuana dispensaries flourish. Cannabis can be smoked or inhaled; taken orally in pill, food, or oil form; taken sublingually; or taken rectally by suppository. Many physicians do not recommend that marijuana be smoked or vaped given possible impurities and effects on lungs that would be less likely with inhalation or drops. The most common cannabis-derived cannabinoids are tetrahydrocannabinol (THC) and cannabidiol (CBD). THC is the component of marijuana that causes the "high." THC alters perception and psychomotor performance. The CBD formulations have little THC and are less likely to cause changes in perceptions.

In the medically ill, CBD has been found to be helpful for treating many maladies, as shown in Box 4.8. It is useful for treating pain, insomnia, anxiety, spasticity, and even epilepsy. It can also help with nausea and with weight loss by stimulating a person's appetite. In particular, it has been helpful for chronic pain and neuropathic pain syndromes and also neurological disorders such as the tremors of Parkinson's disease, fibromyalgia, endometriosis, and interstitial

---

Box 4.8 USES OF CANNABIS IN THE MEDICALLY ILL

- Pain relief
- Insomnia
- Relieve anxiety
- Increase appetite and decrease nausea
- Decrease gastric upset with Crohn's disease
- Decrease tremors related to Parkinson's disease

---

cystitis. In addition, it may improve symptoms of Crohn's disease and irritable bowel syndrome.[3] For patients who use cannabis regularly, withdrawal can upset sleep patterns.

Adverse effects of cannabis include memory and executive function deficits and possibly an increased risk of a psychotic episode. High doses in some patients can cause anxiety and panic symptoms, and chronic use can increase the risk of depression (Box 4.9).

Box 4.9 SIDE EFFECTS OF CANNABIS/CBD IN THE
MEDICALLY ILL

- Mental slowness
- Impaired reaction times
- Increased anxiety
- Withdrawal (about 48 hours to one week after stopping regular use)
  - Irritability
  - Anxiety and restlessness
  - Sleep difficulties
  - Aggression

SAFETY CONSIDERATIONS OF SLEEP MEDICATIONS

Potential Contraindications and Drug Interactions

When discussing with a primary prescriber a patient who might benefit from a sleep medication, consider the patient's current level of sedation and any other factors that may influence their degree of sedation, cognitive stability or impairment, respiratory status, and risk for falls, or further impede immobility and urinary or bowel function. Also consider chronic difficulties the patient may have, such as restless legs syndrome or sleep apnea, as well as concomitant substance use and other medications, including OTC medications or supplements used to treat sleep, or centrally acting medications such as opioids, benzodiazepines, and steroids that can have additive or paradoxical effects on the patient. As noted previously, it is helpful to be aware of the patient's liver, kidney and pulmonary functions to ensure that a medication prescribed for sleep does not make another bodily system worse or impair adequate metabolism.

It is also important to note a patient's baseline cognitive status because all sleep medications can influence cognitive functioning, at least in the short term.

UNDERSTANDING THE STRATEGIES OF THE PSYCHO-ONCOLOGY MEDICATION PRESCRIBER

How Psycho-Oncology Prescribers Choose a Sleep Medication

An important consideration in choosing a sleep medication, as is true with other psychotropic medications, is whether any medications helped the patient fall asleep in the past, without side effects (recognizing they were younger and most likely healthier when they took the medication previously). Addressing substance use and proper sleep hygiene techniques is useful because poor sleep behaviors can counter even a good medication. It will be helpful if any concurrent energizing medications can be altered in terms of time of dosing or dose to minimize the negative influence on sleep while not losing overall efficacy.

Younger patients with cancer can often tolerate and benefit from OTC medications. We have found that both younger and older patients are willing to try medical marijuana for sleep and other symptoms. Those who have been comfortable buying their own marijuana may continue to do so. The prescription of controlled substances varies by state, although since the opioid crisis, more states have become stringent about prescriber and pharmacy compliance. Many prescribers therefore try to limit giving controlled substances. Discussions with patients early on about the short-term nature of the prescription in order to minimize the risk of dependence, tolerance, and addiction are worthwhile, along with the recommendation to limit daily use of the sleep medication to a few weeks as an attempt to reset the aberrant sleep pattern. Afterwards, as-needed (prn) prescription of the sleep medication might be helpful, with the possibility of daily doses again for crisis periods.

Prescribers may start with uncontrolled medications such as the sedating antidepressants. If those do not work and the patient is not elderly or cognitively compromised and has little anxiety, the second line of prescription might be the Z drugs or the benzodiazepine temazepam. If anxiety accompanies the sleep disturbance, an intermediate or longer acting benzodiazepine such as lorazepam or clonazepam can be helpful. If the patient has some additional or concurrent muscle spasms, diazepam might be useful. Clonazepam has been found to be helpful for restless leg syndrome. Given the comfort some oncologists have gained prescribing olanzapine for nausea, they are also comfortable prescribing it for sleep disturbances that are accompanied by anxiety or gastric upset. The atypical antipsychotics olanzapine and quetiapine may also be used to induce sleep in hospitalized patients who have anxiety.

Making Sleep Medications Multitask: The Benefits May Offer Twofers

If a patient can obtain more than one benefit from a medication and possibly reduce the number of medications they need to take, they will usually do so. Therefore, an antihistamine is an excellent option to help with sleep in someone who has itching, allergies, or an allergic reaction to another medication. A sedating antidepressant such as mirtazapine can be helpful in someone who needs sleep but also has nausea and/or gastric upset (recall that mirtazapine does not commonly cause gastric side effects). The benzodiazepines can promote sleep and relieve anxiety as well. For patients who have nausea and sleep problems, lorazepam can be a welcome twofer. Atypical antipsychotics can provide sleep as well as antianxiety relief and a reprieve from nausea. A patient who has difficulty sleeping and neuropathic pain can get double help from either gabapentin or pregabalin. If the patient also has hot flashes, these medications can benefit three ways. The Z drugs, in contrast, may be the only sleep medications that do not provide twofers (or threefers).

CASE: BILL

Bill has kidney cancer and was taking an immunotherapy medication that caused liver toxicity for which he is receiving high-dose steroids. Although he used marijuana to fall asleep prior to his cancer, he has avoided it lately, fearing a negative effect on his cancer. He has tried the calming and sleep hygiene approaches you have taught him, but he says the awakening effect on him by the steroids and the sense of anguish make him feel defeated. He has no suicidal ideation but wants more immediate help because he feels like he is going crazy. You have made a referral to a psychiatrist, but the patient cannot get an appointment for 3 weeks and he does not believe he can wait that long. You and Bill call his oncology team together and discuss the possibility of a sedating atypical antipsychotic to counter the revving effects of the steroids.

SUMMARY

Sleep problems are common in cancer patients. Reviewing sleep hygiene techniques, utilizing cognitive–behaviorally oriented interventions specially designed for insomnia, and sometimes medications are indicated.

When medications are prescribed, they need to be considered carefully in the context of other medications and medical conditions, used for short periods of time, and monitored carefully. As we have seen with other psychopharmacologic interventions in the cancer setting, the non-prescriber and non-psycho-oncologist often have the opportunity to inquire with a prescriber or the primary care team about the use of a psychotropic medication. Non-prescribers can then help the primary team or prescriber monitor the patient for effectiveness and side effects.

NOTES

1. Liu L, Ancoli-Israel S. Sleep Disturbances in Cancer. *Psychiatr Ann.* 2008;38(9):627–634. doi:10.3928/00485713-20080901-01
2. https://www.psychiatry.org/patients-families/sleep-disorders/what-are-sleep-disorders#:~:text=In%20primary%20care%2C%2010%2D20,the%20criteria%20for%20insomnia%20disorder. Accessed 9-1-2020.
3. https://www.health.harvard.edu/blog/medical-marijuana-2018011513085. Accessed 9-3-2020.

Chapter 5

Medications for Fatigue

INTRODUCTION

Cancer-related fatigue is extremely common and can be debilitating.[1-4] Up to 80% of people with cancer complain of significant fatigue at some point. Hearing a person say, "I have no energy" or "I feel like a drained-out dish rag all day long" gives you some sense about what is happening or how distressed someone feels. Additional statements we have heard from patients about their fatigue are listed in Box 5.1. Distressing fatigue can be an isolated experience or can be related to various psychiatric or medical causes, such as significant depression, frequent intense anxiety or panic attacks, as well as sleep disturbances, pain, electrolyte or hormonal abnormalities, and wide-ranging medications and substances. In fact, it is not unusual for fatigue to have multiple etiologies. Non-prescribers can learn the various physiological and metabolic causes of fatigue, increasing their awareness of and alertness to side effects of various medications that might be investigated and corrected by the primary clinician or oncologist. Identifying opportunities to supplement nonpharmacologic therapies with an activating medication can improve a patient's quality of life and joy in living. Understanding the indications,

Box 5.1 ANALYZING FATIGUE: WHAT SOME PEOPLE WITH
CANCER SAY

"I'm tired."

"I feel tired all the time."

"I never feel rested or refreshed, even when I wake up in the
morning."

"I'm exhausted for 3 days after chemotherapy and then I
perk up."

"I feel great for a couple of days after chemotherapy, probably from the steroids they give me, and then I crash for
a few days."

"It's hard to keep my eyes open when I try to read or watch
a movie."

contraindications, and potential side effects of activating agents to
treat fatigue in cancer patients is an important contribution of the
non-prescribing clinician.

As with pain assessment, clinicians emphasize that we must
take patients at their subjective word. However, as with pain,
investigating what is going on is important if we are to provide
relief.

Fatigue can be monitored by self-report. Daily logs such as the
one shown **below**, that track pain or other physical distress such as
gastric upset, anxiety, mood, sleep, fluid and food intake, and irritability can be helpful to isolate associated factors and thus potential
mediators of fatigue. Documenting what activities were attempted
and to what extent they were completed at different times of the

day may identify problematic patterns that can be remediated. Whether the fatigue is primary or secondary to another cause, providing relief can be difficult. As discussed with regard to treating delirium, regulating or fixing the underlying cause of fatigue, if possible, makes sense. The prescribing team can address the underlying causes of fatigue while offering a medication to enhance energy, as discussed with regard to treating depression and anxiety. Energy, fatigue and concentration may be improved by correcting electrolyte irregularities; optimizing hematocrit and hemoglobin in anemia; and improving thyroid, cardiac, neurological, or pulmonary function. But sometimes these parameters cannot be improved sufficiently to provide the desired "get up and go" patients crave to live a more quality-filled life as they deal with cancer or cancer treatment.

Mood/Physical Status Chart

Time	Monday	Tuesday	Wednesday	Thursday	Friyday	Saturday
AM						
MID-DAY						
PM						

Indicate:
*tearfulness *anxiety *sleep *depressed mood *pain *energy *appetite *cocentration
*List as "ok" or "not ok", or on a scale of 0–10
*List possible triggers to problematic symptoms
Also Indicate: good/enjoyable activities

RISK FACTORS FOR FATIGUE IN CANCER PATIENTS

The risk factors for fatigue in people with cancer can be varied, straightforward, or appear to come out of nowhere. Assessing risk factors is important in order to implement proper and successful interventions. People who are less active because of their treatments risk atrophy and weakness of muscles, which may induce fatigue. Many medical conditions, in addition to treatments for different illnesses including cancer, can drain a person's sense of vitality. Some of the causes are listed in Box 5.2. The spectrum between vitality and severe exhaustion or debilitation is quite broad. Thus, determining an individual's energy level, and changing quality of lethargy and stamina over time, can help pinpoint the origins of a person's fatigue. This investigative process can also identify fluctuations, instigating factors, and mitigating factors throughout a day or week, potentially leading to nonpharmacologic and medicinal interventions if needed.

Box 5.2 CAUSES OF FATIGUE IN CANCER PATIENTS

- Primary fatigue problem (not related to an identifiable cause)
- Insufficient physical activity
- Medical comorbidities (i.e., suboptimal cardiac, endocrine, electrolyte, neurological, or pulmonary functioning)
- Medication side effects, polypharmacy, or substance use
- Major psychiatric syndromes (e.g., major depressive disorder, bipolar disorder, generalized anxiety disorder)

Recall from Chapter 1 that we can try to distinguish whether a person is experiencing a significant major depressive episode, with fatigue as one of a cluster of depressive symptoms, from someone who is sad because they feel too tired to do more activities that they would ordinarily like to do by asking, "If we could get you a pill to give you energy, what would you like to do?" The person who is very depressed might shrug their shoulders and say, "I have no idea. What's the point?" The person who is demoralized because of fatigue might say, after giving you a quizzical look, "Well, it would be nice to get out to the park or be able to spend more time with my grandchildren." The latter patient may benefit from an activating agent or a psychostimulant, rather than a general antidepressant.

ALGORITHM FOR ESTABLISHING FATIGUE IN CANCER PATIENTS

The following algorithm highlights a method for determining whether a medication may be helpful for complaints of fatigue:

> Subjective complaint of fatigue

+

> Insufficient behavioral activation because of fatigue

+

> A sleep disturbance cannot be treated adequately

OR

> A major psychiatric disorder when treated does not relieve fatigue

OR

Any fatiguing medications cannot be adjusted and corrected

OR

Any medical causes of fatigue are addressed but do not fix fatigue

=

Fatigue that may be improved pharmacologically

CHALLENGES OF DIAGNOSING FATIGUE IN THE ELDERLY WITH CANCER

People who are elderly or frail are more at risk for fatigue as they go through cancer treatment. Dr. Jimmie Holland, who is considered the architect of the field of psycho-oncology, used to quote Bette Davis when speaking about growing older: "Aging ain't for sissies." Holland understood this from her patients, as well as from her own experience living until almost age 90 years. The decline of different bodily systems takes a toll on emotional and physical well-being, and it takes a degree of mental toughness, acceptance, ingenuity, and resilience to keep moving, and to slow the process of slowing down, and prevent further collateral damage.

When older patients complain that "aging stinks," we often agree and reply "but the alternative [of death] is worse. Let's try to improve how you feel."

INTRODUCING: MR. ATHENS

Mr. Athens is a 73-year-old man with metastatic prostate cancer who is seeing you for supportive therapy to help cope with his cancer diagnosis. He has always been in good physical shape, exercising 5 days a week at the gym. Since going on androgen deprivation therapy (ADT) for his prostate cancer, he has felt sluggish and does not feel like going to the gym anymore because he cannot do the same hefty exercises he used to perform. In fact, he delayed taking the hormonal therapy because he feared losing his testosterone, feeling weak, and looking out of shape. Eventually, his wife convinced him that being alive was more important than how he looked. But his fatigue frustrated him. The behavioral and cognitive interventions you discussed succeeded in getting Mr. Athens to the gym. Although his energy has improved somewhat in the past month, he is still frustrated and does not want to go out socially because of his fatigue. You suggest he speak with his primary care doctor or oncologist about an activating agent or psychostimulant.

MEDICAL LOOK-ALIKES FOR FATIGUE

Fatigue can be a great chameleon of multiple psychological and medical syndromes listed in Box 5.3. This diagnostic quandary

---

Box 5.3 FATIGUE CAN BE THE CAUSE OR THE RESULT:
A MEDICAL CHAMELEON

- Significant depression
- Intense or steady anxiety or panic symptoms
- Endocrine abnormalities (i.e., hypothyroid, adrenal insufficiency)
- Anemia
- Cardiovascular problems
- Pulmonary insufficiency
- Pain
- Electrolyte abnormalities
- Neurological disorders
- Medications and substances

---

makes identification of potential solutions complicated. Cancer-related fatigue can lead to worsening of already existing syndromes, or be secondary to other medical entities. Non-prescribers are an integral component of the oncology team, providing, often in separate time and space from the oncologist, important observations and assessments. Nurses during vital sign checks, psychotherapists in counseling sessions or when assessing family or home conditions, occupational or physical therapists while helping patients improve coordination and strength, and even clergy and other ancillary supports who hear patients' concerns and are asked to improve patients' daily living and function, can provide pertinent insights and help identify pieces to the fatigue puzzle. A multidisciplinary approach may lead to enough improvement to tip the balance in favor of better quality of life for patients.

CASE: MR. ATHENS

Mr. Athens sees his primary care doctor, who performs a thyroid function test and finds that Mr. Athens is slightly hypothyroid. Although Mr. Athens is upset by yet another medical problem with which he must deal, he believes that at least he has a fix. But 6 weeks after starting thyroxine, he tells you he is still fatigued. His demoralization seems to be worsening. In fact, the clinician in you may also be getting demoralized at this point. What do you do?

ASK, BECAUSE THEY MAY NOT TELL; TELL, BEFORE THEY ASK

When patients complain about feeling tired, you can ask them to describe their energy levels at different times of the day using the daily log mentioned previously. A 0–10 visual analog scale can be monitored in the mornings, afternoons, and evenings for a week or two at a time. Ask patients to note what else is going on at the time in terms of other physical symptoms (e.g., pain, nausea, and dizziness), cognitively, and emotionally (e.g., mood, irritability, and anxiety). It can be self-defeating and demoralizing for patients to attempt to accomplish activities such as paying bills, exercising, or performing pleasurable activities during low-energy periods. How they answer the previous questions, and the information reflected in the chart, may point to more appropriately targeted therapeutic suggestions. It can be helpful to perform baseline and periodic cognitive screening exams to monitor the course and association of concentration with other variables such as fatigue, mood and pain.

NONPHARMACOLOGICAL TREATMENTS FOR FATIGUE

Significant symptoms of fatigue can be addressed with nonpharmacological means by non-prescribers and prescribers alike before or during pharmacologic interventions. Nonpharmacological treatments for fatigue, highlighted in Box 5.4, include increasing physical activity and exercise, physical or occupational therapy to improve deconditioning, increasing psychosocial support, addressing poor sleep habits, educating about nutritional deficiencies and poor activity scheduling, assessing the impact of substance use on energy levels, and using cognitive–behaviorally oriented therapy, mindfulness meditation, and other complimentary therapies. Even small incremental increases in activity can be beneficial to turning the tide against fatigue, although it may take time. It may even help a person get to a new horizon of "this is good enough" even though it falls short of fantastic or past performance. It is difficult to get someone who is feeling "washed out" to accept the notion that pushing themselves to walk strengthens muscles and the cardiovascular system in ways that will help the patient reverse and overcome fatigue. "Start low

Box 5.4 NONPHARMACOLOGICAL TREATMENTS FOR FATIGUE

Education

- Nutrition: Understand foods that energize and those that may devitalize
- Scheduling: Take advantage of higher energy periods for activities requiring some drive
- Sleep hygiene

Cognitive–Behaviorally Oriented Therapy

- Behavioral activation: Improve deconditioning and focus with Physical Therapy and Occupational Therapy
- Cognitive reframes to address all-or-none or catastrophic thinking
- Develop an attitude of "something is better than nothing" and "seeing the glass as half full."

Mindfulness Meditation

- Useful to maintain and optimize wakeful periods
- Better appreciate the body's need to rest

Integrative Medicine

- Acupuncture
- Massage
- Other complimentary therapies

and go slowly" works just as well for physical exercise as for dosing medications. And "something is better than nothing" and the Nike slogan of "Just Do It" often help motivate people to get going when they do not feel like doing so, and to perhaps experience the benefits of seeing "the glass half full". It can take weeks of increased activity before patients may experience improved energy, just as it can take weeks before antidepressants relieve severe depression. So ongoing monitoring and realistic encouragement from all clinicians are vital.

MEDS FOR HEADS

Understanding the Strategies of the Psycho-Oncology Medication Prescriber

When the cause of cancer-related fatigue cannot be corrected, or the benefits of sedating medications for pain outweigh their fatiguing side effects, and nonpharmacological interventions are insufficient, medications can be tried to improve the symptoms of physical and cognitive fatigue. These medications include wakefulness agents, psychostimulants, and activating antidepressants. There are few choices, but an understanding of them will help any clinician care better for their patients. You may recognize some of these medications, as do patients, as medications that are used to treat attention-deficit/hyperactivity disorder (ADHD).

We Do Not Fully Know How Activating or Stimulant Medications Work for Fatigue

These medications appear to increase the availability of dopamine, norepinephrine, and serotonin, as discussed for the antidepressant medications, in particular brain synapses, leading to improved focus, decreased impulsivity, and improved energy.

The data on the benefits of wakefulness agents or psychostimulants for cancer related fatigue[5,6] and cognitive slowing in cancer patients are inconsistent, and to date there are no approved medications for cancer-related fatigue. Therefore, our discussion is couched in the disclosure of discussing off-label use of these medications and caution should be used when discussing potential benefits and downsides of using stimulant medications. But as mentioned previously, fatigue that interferes with quality of life can arise from multifactorial causes and can be complicated to diagnose appropriately. The prudent use of these medications in many patients can be safe and their benefits maximized to provide more energy and clarity to enjoy life events and, it is hoped, to propel more behavioral activation, participation in physical therapy or rehabilitation, and cancer treatment. Therefore, as indicated in other chapters, if the potential benefit might outweigh the potential risk, it can be helpful to have discussions with patients and cancer survivors about the benefits and side effects—yes, the pearls and potholes—of medications that can improve quality of life. These discussions may illuminate whether the criteria for an appropriate jeopardy-worthy balance is met for that person.

THE MEDS — JUST THE NAMES

Antidepressants

Bupropion (Wellbutrin)

Fluoxetine (Prozac)

Wakefulness Agents

Modafinil (Provigil)

Armodafinil (Nuvigil)

Psychostimulants

Methylphenidate (Ritalin, Metadate)

Dexmethylphenidate (Focalin)

Dextroamphetamine (Dexedrine)

Mixed amphetamine salts (Adderall)

These medications are often prescribed in immediate-release formulations to quickly provide increased energy and cognitive clarity. However, to avoid the overshoot side effects of anxiety and restlessness, and to prolong the daylong effectiveness of the medications, we sometimes suggest long-acting or slow-release formulations.

WILL THE SYMPTOMS OF FATIGUE TIP A PRESCRIBER TO SUGGEST AN ACTIVATING OR STIMULANT MEDICATION?

Getting a sense of the quality, severity, and duration of a patient's fatigue as elucidated in Box 5.5, as well as the temporal variables of the fatigue, overall medical circumstances of the patient, and the degree

---

Box 5.5 QUESTIONS THAT MAY LEAD TO A REFERRAL FOR A
MEDICATION FOR FATIGUE

How long has the fatigue been lasting?

Is fatigue present every day for most of the day?

Does rest or activation make the fatigue improve?

How severe is the fatigue upon awakening?

How severe is the fatigue through the morning? The afternoon? The evening?

Does caffeine have any effect on the fatigue?

How might the fatigue be related to the patient's overall and current medical situation?

Does the fatigue include slowed concentration or clouded attention?

Does the patient have trouble sitting and reading for more than a short period of time?

---

to which fatigue interferes with an acceptable quality of life, will give a prescriber a good sense of the potential benefit of an activating or stimulant medication. If caffeine improves a patient's energy, but not enough, or if caffeine does not help and there are no changeable medical or medication conditions, or medical contraindications for using a particular agent in a patient, a stimulant may be worth trying.

MYTHS THAT HINDER PATIENTS FROM TAKING ACTIVATING MEDICATIONS OR STIMULANTS

The history of psychostimulants comes with baggage. As with other controlled substances, there is a potential for dependence, tolerance, and addiction. The "uppers" of the 1960s were part of the drug culture in which many people used them just to feel differently, and they were sometimes used as antidotes for other substances that slowed people down. They are also used to help high school and college students stay alert at night to study for examinations. The psychostimulants are also known as diet pills, yet people with cancer may already have a problem maintaining their weight. For many decades, the psychostimulant medications have been a hallmark of treating children with ADHD. It is not easy to see the indication for a medication that treats ADHD when you are dealing with cancer and cancer treatment, especially when there is no formal indication for prescription. Accurate information about these medications and potential benefits of monitored treatment will allay fears of becoming addicted, or of losing weight that a patient cannot afford to lose.

THE MEDESCORT GUIDE

The Short List of Benefits of Stimulating Medications Should Not Be Minimized

Prescribers who are familiar with the vagaries of palliative care and cancer care are comfortable describing to patients the benefits of improved energy and focus. They can describe clinical observations that have seen stimulants in the medically ill often lead to moderate weight gain, perhaps because they facilitate increased activity that may increase the energy requirements, mood, and perhaps interest in eating and consequently improve the appetite of a patient. These medications have even been tolerated in patients with brain tumors who benefit from increased cognitive clarity and energy. As noted in Chapter 1, stimulant medications are relatively fast acting and do not take weeks or months to work if they are indeed going to work. They can be started along with antidepressants to improve the fatigue of depression before the antidepressants have time to be effective. In addition, activating and psychostimulant medications can be very helpful for improving mood, energy, and cognitive clarity in patients

Table 5.1 Activating Antidepressants Used in
the Cancer Setting

Medication	Starting Daily Dose	Non-Psychiatrist Sky View Focus
Bupropion (Wellbutrin)	100 mg SR; 75 mg IR	Can cause anxiety, irritability, and insomnia; contraindicated in those with history of seizure disorders
Fluoxetine (Prozac)	20 mg	Can cause anxiety, irritability, and insomnia; gastric upset

IR, immediate release; SR, sustained release.

who are depressed as they near the end of life and may not have the time to wait for an antidepressant to become effective.

Activating Antidepressants

Bupropion and fluoxetine are the most consistently energizing antidepressants and are described in Table 5.1. As with other antidepressants, both can precipitate anxiety for some, or manic episodes in people with bipolar proclivities. The early activating properties of these medications might be considered side effects and not a function of their antidepressant benefits. Bupropion is highly dopaminergic, which is why it is used to help people stop smoking. It shares some properties with the psychostimulants, which are discussed later. If a patient gets an energizing effect from bupropion, it can be used on an as-needed basis and not necessarily daily. The immediate-release format might have more energizing impact than the slow-release format, although it is also more likely to cause anxiety and a frustrating on–off feeling, leaving a patient feeling suddenly tired after a short burst of energy, as can happen with short-acting psychostimulants.

Wakefulness Agents

Modafinil and armodafinil promote wakefulness, although the mechanism for this effect is still not completely clear. These wakefulness agents, highlighted in Table 5.2, are believed to have effects on several neurotransmitter systems in the brain, mainly in those areas of the brain that regulate sleep, wakefulness, and alertness. These medications are indicated for those who have energy deficits due to a sleep disorder such as sleep apnea and narcolepsy or fatigue related to multiple sclerosis. They are also indicated for pilots who

Table 5.2 Wakefulness Agents

Agent	Starting Dose	Non-Psychiatrist Sky View Focus
Modafinil (Provigil)	50–100 mg or prn	These medications are usually well tolerated. Both can cause anxiety, irritability, and insomnia. They can interact with liver enzymes to cause drug interactions. Hypertension and cardiac arrhythmias must be monitored, although these are less common than with psychostimulants.
Armodafinil (Nuvigil)	50–150 mg	

must fly long distances and need to stay alert for safety reasons and for people who work night shifts and have uncommon sleep–wake cycles. They have not been approved for cancer-related fatigue. They are believed to be gentler stimulants than the psychostimulants; thus, they are potentially a good first step to treating fatigue. However, because there is no formal indication for these medications to treat cancer-related fatigue, some insurance companies do not reimburse patients for their use.

Psychostimulants

The traditional psychostimulants include the amphetamines and methylphenidate. A sky view focus on these medications is shown in Table 5.3. As noted previously, these medications

Table 5.3 Psychostimulants

Psychostimulants	Starting Dose	Sky View Focus
Shorter Acting		
Methylphenidate, dexmethylphenidate (Ritalin, Focalin)	1.25–5 mg in the a.m. and/or early afternoon	Psychostimulants can improve energy, concentration, and appetite.
Dextroamphetamine (Dexedrine)	May be used on an as-needed	These medications can lower seizure threshold; they can
Mixed amphetamine salts (Adderall)	basis	cause anxiety, irritability, restlessness, and insomnia.
		Interactions with liver enzymes causing drug interactions are possible but rare; charts should be checked.
		Observe for hypertension and cardiac arrhythmias; tics, paranoid ideation, or mania.
Longer Acting		
Metadate CD; Concerta; Vyvanse Adderall XR and others		Check literature for dosing (usually less frequent than shorter acting stimulants)— Dosages should be assessed per individual needs.

are better known to treat children and adults with ADHD, although in the past they were known as diet pills and "uppers." The psychostimulants heighten concentration, clarity, and attention so that a person can focus on one activity, such as reading, writing an essay, or studying piano, for longer periods of time. These benefits are seen in the cancer setting as well. Patients with chemotherapy-related cognitive changes find they focus better and longer with a psychostimulant. Stimulants do not necessarily fill all the gaps of cognitive deficits such as impaired multitasking or serial tasking. If attention is improved, people may feel as if their memory is improved too because there is a better chance of enhanced attention to things they might want to remember. These patients may record information in their minds better so that they can have a sharpened sense of recall—although they might describe this as having better memory or less forgetfulness, rather than improved attention. In essence, without the proper tools to focus attention, it is difficult to record information efficiently or effectively. When we do not pay attention, new information is not planted in the brain in the first place, in order to be able to recall it later. Without recording information, it will be difficult to recall it. Cancer, cancer treatment, and aging can all diminish attention abilities and multi- or serial-tasking skills that people had when they were younger and healthier. Psychostimulants can heighten focus sometimes just by improving energy and alertness levels. Men with prostate cancer who had fatigue from ADT have been shown to be more energized while taking a psychostimulant over time.[7]

CASE: MR. ATHENS

You suggested to Mr. Athens that he ask his oncologist whether his fatigue can be treated. He tells his oncologist that he is considering discontinuing hormonal therapy because his current condition is not a life worth living. His oncologist examines Mr. Athens for other possible causes of fatigue, noting his recent treatment for hypothyroidism. When offered an activating antidepressant, Mr. Athens becomes upset and says, "That's what my daughter took for ADHD problems and depression. That's not for me doc. I'm just really washed out; I just need some energy." The oncologist obtains an electrocardiogram and finds that Mr. Athens has no arrhythmia and sees from his vital signs that all of the exercise Mr. Athens has done during his life has helped keep his blood pressure and heart rate in an excellent zone. Given that Mr. Athens has no history of seizures and no arrhythmia, the oncologist offers methylphenidate concluding that Mr. Athens can tolerate a psychostimulant. Although Mr. Athens does not want to taking any medication that will artificially energize him, especially one whose name starts with "psycho," he recognizes that for many years he has often had two large cups of coffee each day but "They just don't help the way they used to."

Making Activating or Stimulant Medications Multitask: The Benefits of Twofers

As noted previously, fatigue can be experienced physically and cognitively. If either or both of these are improved, a patient may be more satisfied at home, school, or work and thus be more adherent to, and tolerant of, behavioral activation, as well as occupational, physical, or cognitive therapy schedules and arduous cancer regimens.

TOPICS TO ADDRESS WITH PATIENTS, SO THEY CAN ASK THEIR PRESCRIBER

The non-prescriber can help set the stage for a more successful outcome when the use of activating or stimulant medications is addressed with the prescriber. Non-prescribers can help the patient clarify what fatigue or tiredness means to them and how it is impacting their lives. They can assist in developing a clear history and day-by-day map of the patient's fatigue that includes the possible modifiers and consequences of their fatigue. Patients will also benefit by asking about whether they have potential contraindications to a stimulant medication either because of a chronic or acute medical condition or because of current medications that might negatively interact with a stimulant medication. Questions will arise about whether there is a history of a seizure disorder or about a cardiac arrhythmia or hypertension that might worsen if severe or not well controlled.

POTENTIAL POTHOLES OF ACTIVATING OR STIMULANT TREATMENT

Activating Antidepressants

Bupropion is contraindicated in people with a history of seizures or bulimia. As with all stimulating medications, it can overshoot into feelings of anxiety, restlessness, and lead to difficulty sleeping. Fluoxetine, the first selective serotonin reuptake inhibitor released in the 1980s, is long acting, so if a patient obtains an energized effect, this can last much of the day. It can lead to anxiety and insomnia if the energizing side effect overshoots its intended goal. Compared to bupropion, it is less consistent as an energizing medication, so it is not often used for this purpose. Both medications, regardless of their primary purpose, can have gastric upset side effects including nausea, bloating, and change in bowel habits.

Wakefulness Agents

All wakefulness agents and stimulants can increase heart rate and blood pressure. Modafinil and armodafinil do not usually require cardiology clearance; however, it is recommended if a patient has a history of hypertension, arrhythmias, or other cardiac problems. Any wakefulness agent, such as caffeine, can increase heart rate. This can be problematic in patients with arrhythmias or unstable heart rates.

Both modafinil and armodafinil are metabolized through the cytochrome P450 3A4 protein processing system; they can interact with many other medications. Some of these interactions can decrease the activity of a cancer-treating medication, so awareness of this potential pothole is important.

Psychostimulants

Sometimes too much of a good thing is not good. Attempts to improve energy and clarity can lead to anxiety, restlessness, irritability, or insomnia. Longer term side effects can include muscular tics, paranoia, and mania. These medications can be abused, sold, or diverted, and they can become addictive. Many will develop dependence and need to be weaned off when they want to stop the medication. These medications need to be monitored by prescribers and non-prescribers for proper usage and effectiveness.

CASE: MR. ATHENS

Mr. Athens comes to see you with his wife. He seems pleased that he has more energy since taking methylphenidate and he says he is willing to accept that he does not sleep as much—he thinks this may be due to the hot flashes he has been getting from his ADT, but his wife complains that he has been more irritable, snapping at her over the smallest of issues. Mr. Athens agrees with this but says he has always had a short temper. You review communication strategies with them but also suggest that they speak with the oncologist to determine if a change in the dose of methylphenidate or a change of medication might be indicated.

When they return to see you 3 weeks later, they report that the methylphenidate was changed to modafinil. The patient has less irritability. He has sufficient energy, although it is slightly little less than he had with methylphenidate. He appreciates sleeping better and believes he has enough energy to do the activities that are important to him, and his wife is glad to have a happier husband back.

SUMMARY

Activating antidepressants, wakefulness agents, and the psycho-stimulants are considered off-label usages for cancer-related fatigue. By improving physical energy and cognitive clarity, they have been found to improve the quality of life of many patients who tolerate them. As with other entities described in this book, a careful assessment is suggested to understand whether a psychiatric or medical cause for the fatigue can be reversed, whether a nonpharmacologic intervention is indicated and appropriate, and when to request an assessment for a medication prescription. As with other psychotropic medications, there can be side effects, so a careful discussion with the patient about risks and benefits is indicated, as well as ongoing monitoring by all providers.

NOTES

1. Wagner L, Cella D. Fatigue and cancer: causes, prevalence and treatment approaches. *Br J Cancer.* 2004;91:822–828.
2. Ahlberg K, Ekman T, Gaston-Johansson F, Mock V. Assessment and management of cancer-related fatigue in adults. *Lancet.* 2003;362:640–650.
3. Stone P, Richards M, A'Hern R, Hardy J. A study to investigate the prevalence, severity and correlates of fatigue among patients with cancer in comparison with a control group of volunteers without cancer. *Ann Oncol.* 2000;11:561–567.
4. Vogelzang NJ, Bretibart W, Cella D, et al. Patient, caregiver and oncologist perceptions of cancer-related fatigue: results of a tripart assessment survey. The Fatigue Coalition. *Semin Hematol.* 1997 Jul;34(3 Suppl):4–12.
5. Breitbart W, Rosenfeld B, Kaim M, Funesti-Esch J. A randomized, double blind placebo-controlled trial of psychostimulants for the treatment of fatigue in ambulatory patients with HIV disease. *Arch Intern Med.* 2001;161:411–420.
6. Yennurajalingam S, Bruera E. Review of clinical trials of pharmacologic interventions for cancer-related fatigue: focus on psychostimulants and steroids. *Cancer J.* 2014;20(5):319–324. doi:10.1097/PP).0000000000000069.
7. Roth AJ, Nelson C, Rosenfeld B, et al. Methylphenidate for fatigue in ambulatory men with prostate cancer. *Cancer.* 2010 Nov 1;116(21):5102–5110. doi:10.1002/cncr.25424.

Conclusion

This book contains the essence of years of experience caring for people with cancer and being supervised by many who trailblazed the specialty of psycho-oncology. Our goal was to provide a road map with enough directions for non-prescribers and prescribers alike who care for people with cancer to improve pharmacologic treatment of distress, but not to get too bogged down with too many academic references. There is a suggested reading section for those who want to learn more. This guide is designed to be a handy reference for clinicians of all disciplines who work in cancer settings, as well as ancillary specialists in the cancer world, including, but not limited to, clergy, patient representatives, and clerks who interact with patients and family members.

The art of diagnosing depression, anxiety, delirium, insomnia, and fatigue in cancer care is not always straightforward. We have laid out pearls and potholes to assist uncovering the varied and sometimes hidden sources of that distress; to be aware of which syndromes may be amenable to a psychopharmacologic intervention; to know when to refer to prescribers or specialists in psycho-oncology; to hone communication techniques that will facilitate a patient's care; to learn about the strategies psycho-oncologists use to choose the right medications for particular situations; and to recognize how to watch for the benefits and side effects of those medications, which if not understood by all providers and patients can lead to premature discontinuation of potential helpful remedies or untoward side effects.

We do not believe medications are the best choice for all symptoms of physical, psychological, or existential distress in people with cancer. However, medications should also not be shunned out of hand. The sum of these parts often provides for a richer, more coherent whole person as a cancer journey is navigated. We hope this book empowers all providers to improve the quality of their patients' lives and thereby make their own work more rewarding and meaningful. We tried to achieve a common denominator of informational and educational, while maintaining practical usefulness. Our MedEscort guide will be useful to copy and carry in your white coat pocket when working on an inpatient medical unit or to keep on your desk when in your office. Our pearls and potholes will help a patient's overt or disguised symptoms jump off the page to help you identify a problem and potential solution. We also note prescription twofers, where a medication may have more than one benefit because of useful side effects, as well as off-label uses for some medications, whereby medications can be used for purposes not originally intended but useful nonetheless. We hope this will be a convenient helpful guide for senior and novice practitioners, non-providers and providers, alike.

SUGGESTED READINGS

Breitbart W (Ed.). *Psycho-Oncology 4th Edition.* Oxford University Press, In press.

Breitbart W, Alici A (Eds). *Psychosocial Palliative Care.* Oxford University Press, 2014.

Caruso C, Grassi L, Nanni MG, Riba M. Psychopharmacology in psycho-oncology. *Curr Psychiatry Rep* 2013;15:393. doi:10.1007/s11920-013-0393-0

Grassi L, Riba M (Eds). *Psychopharmacology in Oncology and Palliative Care A Practical Manual.* Springer, 2014.

Chochinov HM, Breitbart W, *Handbook of Psychiatry in Palliative Medicine, 2nd ed.* New York: Oxford University Press, 2009.

Holland J, Golant M, Greenberg DB, Hughes MK, Levenson JA, Loscalzo MJ, Pirl WF (Eds.). *Psycho-Oncology: A Quick Reference on the Psychosocial Dimensions of Cancer Symptom Management (APOS Clinical Reference Handbooks), 2nd Edition.* Oxford University Press, 2015.

Holland JC, Weiss Wiesel T, Nelson CJ, Roth AJ, Alici Y (Eds.). *Geriatric Psycho-Oncology: A Quick Reference on the Psychosocial Dimensions of Cancer Symptom Management (APOS Clinical Reference Handbooks), 1st Edition.* Oxford University Press, 2015.

Roth AJ. *Managing Prostate Cancer: A Guide For Living Better.* Oxford University Press, 2016.

Stern TA, Freudenreich O, Smith FA, Fricchione GL, Rosenbaum JF. *Massachusetts General Hospital Handbook of General Hospital Psychiatry, 7th Edition.* Elsevier 2017.

Thekdi SM, Trinidad A, Roth A. Psychopharmacology in cancer. *Curr Psychiatry Rep.* 2015 Jan;17(1):529.

INDEX

For the benefit of digital users, indexed terms that span two pages (e.g., 52–53) may, on occasion, appear on only one of those pages.

Tables, figures and boxes are indicated by t, f and b following the page number